STRONG WOMEN

STAY SLIM

By the same authors

STRONG WOMEN STAY YOUNG

MIRIAM E. NELSON, PH.D.

with Sarah Wernick, Ph.D.

STRONG WOMEN

STAY SLIM

MENUS AND RECIPES
BY STEVEN RAICHLEN
ILLUSTRATIONS BY WENDY WRAY

AURUM PRESS

The PAR-Q test on page 98, from the 1994 revised version of the Physical Activity Readiness Questionnaire (PAR-Q & YOU), has been reprinted with permission from the Canadian Society for Exercise Physiology, Inc. The PAR-Q & YOU is a copyrighted, pre-exercise screen owned by the Canadian Society for Exercise Physiology.

The Body Mass Index table on page 91 has been adapted with permission from George A. Bray, M.D., copyright © 1988.

The statements in the box on page 94 have been adapted with permission from Anorexia Nervosa and Related Eating Disorders, Inc.

The research described in this book has been funded at least in part with federal funds from the US Department of Agriculture, Agricultural Research Service. The contents of this publication do not necessarily reflect the views or policies of the US Department of Agriculture, nor does mention of trade names, commercial products, or organizations imply endorsement by the US Government.

First published in Great Britain
1999 by Aurum Press Ltd
25 Bedford Square, London WC1B 3AT

First published in the United States 1998
Copyright © 1998 by Miriam E. Nelson, Ph.D., and Sarah Wernick, Ph.D.
Section IV, Menus and Recipes, copyright 1998 by Steven Raichlen
Illustrations by Wendy Wray/Vicki Morgan Associates, NYC

A catalogue record for this book is available from the British Library.
ISBN 1 85410 605 8

1   3   5   7   9   10 8   6   4   2
1999   2001   2003   2002   2000

Printed in Great Britain by Redwood Books, Trowbridge.

For my past and present students

▼   ▼   ▼   ▼

CONTENTS

▼   ▼   ▼   ▼

ACKNOWLEDGEMENTS

▼   ▼   ▼   ▼

This book would not have been possible without the expertise and assistance of many people. I want to thank these individuals for their generous support.

During the research and writing of this book, I was fortunate to have the help of two superb assistants:

Jennifer Layne, M.S., C.S.C.S., my extraordinary research associate, was part of this project from conception to completion. Jennifer helped me identify women to test the programme and discuss their experiences. She worked with me in developing the exercises, and she led the exercise segments of our focus group meetings. I benefited tremendously from her knowledge, experience, and creativity—as well as from her encouragement and support.

Melissa Allen, M.S., R.D., my very talented graduate student and research dietitian, worked with me on the nutrition programme. She was invaluable in the design of the food plan, and she led the nutrition segments of the focus group, working closely with participants. Melissa also located women to test the programme and share their stories. Her expertise, ingenuity, and hard work were greatly appreciated.

I've had enormous help from my colleagues at Tufts University: Ronenn Roubenoff, M.D., Irwin Rosenberg, M.D., Susan Roberts, Sc.D., Jacob Selhub, Ph.D., Jose Ordovas, Ph.D., Jeffrey Blumberg, Ph.D., Carmen Castaneda Sceppa, M.D., Ph.D., Christina Economos, Ph.D., Roger Fielding, Ph.D., Charles Pu, M.D., and Jeanne Goldberg, Ph.D., R.D. These leading scientists shared their expertise and their time, brainstorming the concepts of this programme, updating me on their research, and reviewing chapters of the manuscript as they were written. I've also benefited from the kind assistance of colleagues outside Tufts. Steven Blair, P.E.D., of the Cooper Institute for Aerobics Research in Dallas, Texas, answered my many detailed questions regarding physical activity and health. Eric Poehlman, Ph.D., of the

University of Vermont, provided valuable information about the determinants of energy metabolism.

Julia Robarts, R.D., did a painstaking review of the menus and recipes, to make sure the nutrition information was accurate. I also want to acknowledge the expert assistance of my past research technician, Sharon Bortz, M.S., R.D., who helped to design and lead the pilot research project that inspired this programme. And I'm very grateful to Mike Pimentel, L.A.T.C., C.S.C.S., for his extensive efforts coordinating the photo shoot for the illustrations.

A special thanks to Larry Lindner and the *Tufts University Health & Nutrition Letter* for continuing to bring our research findings to the general public.

For their support, I also want to thank the Brookdale Foundation and the Mary Ingraham Bunting Institute at Radcliffe College, where I am currently a Bunting Fellow.

I'm very grateful to the many people who helped me translate what I've learned in the laboratory into a practical book for women:

I am forever indebted to my collaborator and dear friend, Sarah Wernick, who worked with me day in and day out to get this book written. I am in awe of her talent. She was always able to push me further to develop interesting scientific facts and personal stories for our readers.

I want to thank Steven Raichlen, cookbook author extraordinaire, for his brilliant menus and recipes—proof that healthy can be delicious.

Wendy Wray has graced the pages of this book with her illustrations. I appreciate not only her artistry but also her careful attention to detail.

Toni Burbank, my editor at Bantam, and her associates have been incredibly supportive. Toni is a rare and wonderful editor who is able to find the magical balance between respecting the writer's vision and advocating for the readers' needs. I benefited tremendously from her many helpful suggestions. I also want to give heartfelt thanks to Robin Michaelson, Toni's very able assistant, for all the help she so competently and cheerfully provided.

My literary agent, Wendy Weil, has been an enthusiastic advocate for this book. I'm so grateful for her expertise and her encouragement.

Three talented writers critiqued the manuscript as it became a book. My gratitude to Sally Wendkos Olds, Barbara Sofer, and Anita Bartholemew for their valuable comments and suggestions. Special thanks to my colleague William Lockeretz, Ph.D., who carefully reviewed the entire manuscript for both technical and grammatical accuracy.

Working with women in the laboratory and in our focus groups has been one of the most enjoyable parts of my work. My gratitude to the dedicated volunteers who have so generously given their time to participate in my research. A warm thank-you to the wonderful women in the focus groups who did the exercises, followed the food plan, and gave us helpful feedback: Ruth, Judy, Judith, Dianne, Jane, Batya, Sarah, Nancy, Therese, and Alexandra. For sharing their personal stories, I'm grateful to the women in the focus group, as well as to Susan, Isabel, Martha, Lillian, Diana, Bobbie, Deborah, Denise, Regina, Pat, Sue, Flora, Jill, and Verna.

Thank you to Dorothy Barron, Susan Zellman-Rohrer, Leslie Abad, Felina Mucha-Kangas, Cora Thompson, Carolyn Resendes, Mary Ellen Alonso, Judy Deemys, Yukiyo Iida, and Claudia Wiatr for their assistance with the illustrations and various aspects of the book.

Finally, I want to thank my family and friends for their great encouragement with this project. I especially want to thank my husband, Kin, and my children, Mason, Eliza, and Alexandra, for their continuous love, patience, and support.

I

WEIGHING THE
SCIENTIFIC EVIDENCE

PUTTING NEW MUSCLE

INTO WEIGHT LOSS

From my teens through my twenties, I was always struggling with the same 9 kilograms (20 lb). I didn't eat excessive amounts, but I ate the wrong foods—a lot of sweets. I managed to lose 4.5 kilos (10 lb) through excessive aerobic exercise: I'd go to step class for an hour, then spend 45 minutes on a stair climber. But even that stopped working when I was in my early thirties.

I was determined to lose 4.5 more kilos (10 lb), and I wanted to eat better. So a year and a half ago I began to follow a flexible, healthy diet that I could adapt to my lifestyle. In two months I lost 2 kilos (4½ lb), and I stopped stressing out about food. Then I started strength training, and it made all the difference! I lost those last 2.5 kilos (5 lb), and my figure changed. I'd been pear-shaped—my tops were size 12, but my bottoms were size 16 or 18. Now I can wear size 12 suits. My strength has increased tenfold. I got married a few months ago, and my husband was amazed by what I could lift when we were moving into our new home. He said, "I can't believe how strong you are!"

— Susan

I went through some difficult changes in my life when I turned 40, and gained about 18 kilos (40 lb). I avoided looking in the mirror—I wore huge tanks and covered myself up. Then my picture was in the local newspaper. I was appalled; I didn't recognise myself. I joined a weight-loss class and started doing aerobics, but I was having pain in my knees and hips. It hadn't occurred to me to add strength training until I saw an article about the research at Tufts. I decided to try it.

The results have been a dream come true. I've lost the weight. I feel so much younger; I have so much more energy. I can do things I didn't think were possible. I used to run—I love how it makes me feel. But I'd written that off when I was 35, because my orthopaedist said, "Don't do it if it makes your knees and hips hurt." Now I can run every other day for an hour. Because I feel stronger physically, I feel like a stronger person from a psychological standpoint. My picture was in the paper again recently, and I was quite pleased!

— Isabel

♦ ♦ ♦

I'm a scientist at the Jean Mayer USDA Human Nutrition Research Center on Aging at Tufts University. For the past ten years, our laboratory has studied the health benefits of strength training. My particular research has shown that strengthening exercise can prevent the muscle loss and bone loss that debilitates so many women later in life. Along the way, I've become increasingly excited by another discovery: that strength training is also a remarkably effective aid to weight loss.

You may have read my first book, *Strong Women Stay Young*, which explains the benefits of weight lifting. The book was based on my research, published in the *Journal of the American Medical Association* (*JAMA*), showing that strengthening exercise not only makes women stronger but also builds bone, improves balance and flexibility, and increases energy. I had recruited 40 women who were at risk of muscle and bone loss: they were postmenopausal, sedentary, and not taking hormones. Before they started, I warned the volunteers that they'd have to avoid changes that could confuse our findings: for the next year they could *not* lose weight or begin aerobic exercise.

The women were very conscientious. But they changed anyway—they couldn't help it.

- ◆ Dorothy, who had been wearing size 20, was careful to maintain her weight. But after a few months of strength training, she noticed that her clothing was becoming loose. "I knew I needed a smaller size, so I bought 18s," she says. "Then I had to take them back because I needed 14s and sometimes 12s. My legs and hips became trimmer, and my arms got much more firm."

- ◆ Beth was shapelier, thanks to strength training. "My weight was never out of control, but there was fat in the wrong places," she says. "My inner thigh flab trimmed up, my upper arms got firmer, and I lost my tummy."

- ◆ Flora kept her promise not to start aerobics. But her new strength gave her so much extra energy that she took up ballroom dancing. Says Flora, "My girlfriend kept asking me to come with her, but I used to think the muscles in my calves would bother me. Now I can dance all night."

While this project was going on, my colleagues and I began a pilot study to see whether strength training could prevent muscle and bone loss in another especially vulnerable group: women who were losing weight. Many women are shocked to learn that this is an at-risk category. They assume that when they lose weight the only thing their body burns up is unwanted excess fat. Until recently that's what doctors and scientists believed too. But researchers have taken a closer look and discovered something disturbing: **When women diet, at least 25 to 30 per cent of the weight they shed is not fat, but water, muscle, bone and other lean tissue.** This is true no matter how much protein and calcium their food plan includes. And the faster they lose weight, the larger the proportion that isn't fat.

I had been greatly encouraged by research from the University of Michigan showing that strength training could help women preserve muscle while they lost weight, and I wanted to explore this further. For our pilot study, my colleagues and I put ten overweight women on individually customised food plans designed for slow but steady weight loss. Half of them came to our laboratory twice a week and did strength training; the others just followed the diet.

Our diet-only volunteers lost an average of 5.9 kilos (13 lb) during the study. The women who strength trained lost about the same amount—6 kilos (13 lb 4 oz). But the scale didn't tell the whole story. A dramatic difference emerged when we looked at body composition. Women in the diet-only group had lost an average 1.3 kilos (3 lb) of lean tissue—mainly muscle— along with the fat. In contrast, the women who'd done strength training actually *gained* around 0.5 kilo (1 lb) of lean tissue. So every ounce they lost was fat. Indeed, since the new muscle replaced fat, their total fat loss was 6.6 kilos (14½ lb). They lost 44 per cent more fat than the diet-only group.

Our volunteers were thrilled to find an exercise at which they could excel. They became stronger, fitter, healthier, much more physically active—and were filled with self-confidence. Pat, who lost 13 kilos (28 lb), says:

> *Strength training helped the weight loss a lot. My metabolic rate went up, so I can eat more. I wear a smaller size than if I'd just lost weight and didn't build muscle. My doctor was very happy because my cholesterol and blood pressure went down. I have so much more energy—I feel invigorated. It gives you more self-esteem, a more positive feeling about anything you want to do.*

After *Strong Women Stay Young* was published, I received hundreds of letters, faxes, phone calls, and e-mail messages from readers all over the world. Many of these women found, to their great delight, that strength training had helped them lose weight. Centimetres, as well as kilos, had vanished. The women looked better, felt healthier. Becoming strong had boosted their energy and vitality. Letter after letter spoke of new happiness and self-confidence.

- Diana: *I've only lost 4.5 kilos (10 lb), but people are saying, "You are losing so fast!"*

- Bobbie: *I'm now 42, but I feel like I'm in my twenties! Two years ago I was 4.5 kilos (10 lb) heavier, had constant back pain, and felt slightly depressed. I was walking six kilometres (3½ miles) a day, and thought this was all I should be doing. Then I started weight training, and everything changed. I wish I had discovered this ten years ago. I feel so good! I ski, and I do in-line skating—they were easy to master once I was strong.*

Along with the progress reports came questions:

Should I be doing aerobics too—and if so, how much?
What food should I eat?
Do I need to take a vitamin supplement if I'm losing weight?

I have the great privilege to work at Tufts University, along with dozens of other scientists involved in exciting new research on nutrition, exercise, and health. I discussed the readers' concerns with my colleagues, as well as with some of the many experts from other institutions who visit our laboratories to exchange information. I began to realise how much different specialists have learned about what works for healthy long-term weight loss. What was needed, I became convinced, was a comprehensive programme that would pull together the essential pieces. I wanted to combine new findings about strength training with up-to-date information on nutrition and physical activity. My aim was to come up with a practical programme that would not only help women lose weight permanently but would also become the foundation for a long, healthy, vibrant life. That's why I decided to write *Strong Women Stay Slim*.

THE DESPERATE STRUGGLE

So many women are battling to lose weight—yet they keep getting heavier and heavier. Since 1980 the prevalence of excess weight in American women has jumped by nearly 10 per cent, according to the US Department of Health and Human Services. We don't need government statistics to see the changes as we get older. One woman in five is overweight in her twenties. The problem intensifies during the later reproductive years: more than a third of women aged 30 to 49 weigh too much. But the numbers really soar at menopause. An astonishing 52 per cent of women in their fifties are overweight.

We all know that excess weight endangers health. Overweight triples the normal risk of heart disease and stroke, contributes to diabetes and has even been linked to cancer. Dr C. Everett Koop, the former US Surgeon General, estimates that 300,000 Americans die from excess-weight-related causes each year! And millions of heavy women suffer from associated medical conditions that diminish the quality of their lives—from heartburn to joint pain, to infertility. The burden is emotional as well. Many women are caught in a sad vicious circle: feeling depressed about their weight, seeking consolation in food, gaining more weight, and feeling even worse.

In desperation, some turn to risky medications and fad diets. But it's actually healthier to remain heavy than to lose weight the wrong way. I'm not just talking about the obvious dangers, like life-threatening side effects from drugs or nutritional deficiencies from unbalanced diets. Even the standard "sensible" advice—to eat 1000 to 1200 calories a day—puts women at risk because they lose so much lean tissue along with fat.

Preserving muscle and bone is vitally important for women. We start out with a lot less muscle and bone than men do, so we have a narrower margin of safety. Yet we live longer, so we're much more likely to reach an age where our lives are severely limited by muscular weakness or fragile bones.

But there's a much more immediate reason to be concerned about the loss of lean tissue: the less muscle you have, the harder it is to lose weight and to maintain the loss. Muscle is metabolically active; body fat isn't. So the smaller the proportion of lean tissue in your body, the lower your metabolic rate. To make matters worse, when you lose muscle, you become weaker and have less energy. Consequently you're likely to burn fewer calories through physical activity. If you've ever hit a long plateau during a diet and remained stuck at the same weight despite all your efforts, this could be a reason.

The kind of dieting that leads to muscle loss also sabotages metabolism in another way: by cutting calories too drastically. Nature cleverly designed the human body so we could survive famine. If you put yourself on starvation rations—and for some women even 1200 calories a day is starving—you trigger hormonal shifts that help the body conserve kilojoules instead of burning them. But when you're trying to lose weight, that's the last thing you want! Between the starvation effect and muscle loss, **the wrong diet can reduce your metabolic rate by up to 30 per cent.**

These metabolic changes help explain the all-too-common phen-omenon of "yo-yo" dieting: a woman manages to lose weight—but in the process she undermines herself by depressing her metabolism. Maintaining the loss is a losing battle. She's ravenous all the time; her energy disappears. Eventually she gives in to her hunger and quickly regains.

After one of these discouraging cycles, a woman might console herself with the thought that she's no worse off than when she started her diet. Unfortunately, that's not true. The weight she lost was partly lean tissue, but nearly everything she regained is fat. Because she has less muscle now, it's going to be harder than ever to lose. What's more, repeated bouts of yo-yo dieting increase the risk of heart disease and stroke.

Once scientists and doctors understood the key role of lean tissue in metabolism, they began looking for ways that people could conserve muscle while shedding kilos. The answer turned out to be very simple: strengthening exercise.

THE FAT-FIGHTING POWER OF STRENGTH TRAINING

With strength training, you don't merely lose weight—you give your-self the leaner, healthier body of someone who's naturally slim. The benefits start with muscle and metabolism, but they go even further.

Here's how strength training helps you lose weight forever:

◆ PRESERVES MUSCLE AND BONE AS YOU SHED FAT

I've already explained that women usually lose muscle when they diet. Another disturbing finding of particular concern to women is this: at least seven well-controlled studies have shown that when you diet and lose weight, you lose bone too. A 1994 study done at the Queens Medical Centre in Nottingham, England, studied premenopausal women who dieted for three months. Even though they followed a sensible food plan for modest weight loss (the average was just 3.4 kilos/7½ lb), they lost 1 per cent of their bone mass. That's an alarming change for so short a period in women under age 50, who normally lose no more than half a per cent in an entire year.

We know that strength training can preserve muscle when women are losing weight, and we think that it may help prevent bone loss as well. Several investigators currently are examining this question, and I look forward to seeing their results.

♦ REVS UP YOUR METABOLISM

Have you ever noticed that your male friends and relatives can eat much more than you do without gaining weight? Men really do have a metabolic advantage. But the explanation isn't their hormones, it's their muscles.

Strength training gives your metabolism a boost. You burn calories when you strength train—and you also burn more calories throughout the day when you have more lean tissue. In a study performed in our laboratory, which was published in the *American Journal of Clinical Nutrition,* the combined difference amounted to about 15 per cent. That translates into an extra 300 calories per day for the average woman.

♦ FIRMS AND TIGHTENS, SO YOU LOOK TRIMMER

A kilo of fat is bulkier than a kilo of muscle. So if your weight loss is almost all fat, you'll look trimmer than if you lose lean tissue too. The women in my *JAMA* study all agreed not to lose weight. Nevertheless, many of them dropped one to three sizes because their bodies were more toned.

Nancy, one of the women in the group that tested the programme in this book, reported:

> *The other day I needed a dress for a wedding. My teenage daughter had a navy sheath that was perfect. But I had been size 18 going on size 20, and this was size 16. Also, the dress didn't have sleeves, and I'd never worn anything sleeveless because my arms were always too flabby. I tried it on anyway. My daughter said, "It looks great—your arms aren't flabby at all!" So that's what I wore.*

♦ EASES YOU INTO A MORE PHYSICALLY ACTIVE LIFESTYLE

Becoming more active is not only a tremendous help to weight loss—it's also the key to staying slim. First, you burn extra calories when you move.

Second, your metabolism remains slightly elevated for several hours after exercise. Third, there's evidence that being active helps tame your appetite. Moreover, an active lifestyle conditions your heart and lungs, making you fitter and healthier.

The problem is that many overweight women don't enjoy physical activity—and for good reason. Understandably, they feel self-conscious about pulling on a leotard and joining an exercise class. Even walking has little appeal for someone who's out of shape, especially if her joints ache and she becomes winded in a few minutes.

Strength training makes all the difference. The stronger your muscles, the easier it is to get moving. All the women in my *JAMA* study, as I've mentioned previously, were sedentary and had actually been directed *not* to begin an exercise programme. Nevertheless, these revitalised women spontaneously began walking more, climbing more steps, and selecting more active leisure activities like dancing, hiking and gardening. When we added it all up, after a year of strength training they had become 27 per cent more active! We've now seen similar results in three other studies.

♦ Makes You Healthier

You've heard about weight-loss methods that carry alarming risks—surgery that could shorten your life, pills that might damage your heart. Strength training is different. Instead of risks and side effects, it offers impressive health *advantages.* All women benefit from increased strength. Women over age 40 gain even more, because strength training reverses age-related muscle and bone loss; it even improves balance and flexibility. Indeed, as I'll explain in Chapter 3, strength training is one of the most effective ways to combat osteoporosis and the frailty too often associated with aging.

♦ ♦ ♦

When I was 36, I had a blood clot in my leg. I'm 48 now, and I'm looking towards menopause. I know I'm not a candidate for oestrogen therapy. Strength training is a great alternative.
— *Martha*

♦ ♦ ♦

♦ HELPS YOU FEEL GOOD ABOUT YOURSELF

When I work with women who are strength training, some of the most significant changes I see are emotional. Physical strength is something that women rarely expect of themselves. But when a woman becomes strong, her self-confidence and self-esteem soar. The effect is especially powerful for women who are overweight and sedentary.

Excess weight is a handicap for many forms of exercise—but not for strength training. Indeed, very heavy women are often quite strong. It's always a special joy to watch an overweight woman—someone who may never have succeeded at any physical activity in her entire life—discover that she's not merely capable of lifting weights but actually good at it! Her whole view of herself is transformed.

Over and over, I've seen strength training open the door for weight loss. Dianne, one of the women in the group that helped me refine the programme for this book, isn't sure exactly how much she weighed when she started because her scales don't register above 130 kilos (285 lb). "I guess it was about 153 (335 lb)," she says. Aerobic exercise was out of the question for her—even five minutes of walking left her winded and made her legs ache unbearably. "I wanted to exercise, but how could I? I was a ball of jelly," says Dianne. "Then I read about strength training. Boing! A light went on in my head. Here was something that would bring me to a point where I could be more active."

Dianne became the star of our test group, rapidly graduating from 1.35-kg (3-lb) dumbbells, to 2.25-kg (5-lb), then 3.60-kg (8-lb), 4.50-kg (10-lb), and even 6.80-kg (15-lb) dumbbells for some exercises. Other changes followed. "Strength training gave me an overall sense of wellness, and it snowballed," says Dianne. "I started to eat better within two weeks. I could see myself getting more involved in my own life, being better to myself. I became more active in little ways—instead of sending my daughter upstairs to get my earrings or my watch, I'd go myself. I parked at the far end of the lot when I went to work."

By the end of ten weeks, Dianne had lost more than 16 kilos (35 lb)—and she glowed with vitality. The woman who could barely manage a five-minute walk when she started had joined a gym and was regularly walking 30 minutes on a treadmill. Says Dianne, "It's been a great uplift—I feel so much more positive." I'm thrilled with Dianne's progress so far and look forward to watching her continue.

THE *STRONG WOMEN STAY SLIM* PROGRAMME

The *Strong Women Stay Slim* programme combines the power of strength training with nutritious eating and an active lifestyle. It's not just a weight loss programme; it's a way to become healthier for a lifetime.

EXERCISE YOU CAN DO

Regardless of how much you weigh, you can become active and fit. Instead of starting with aerobic exercise, this programme begins with strength training. There's no huffing and puffing, no special clothes, no getting down on the floor (and struggling to get up again). You'll love the quick results you get with strength training. What a confidence booster!

If you've been sedentary, you'll systematically increase your activity in your third week on the programme. By then you'll be stronger, so moving will be easier and more fun. Over the next eight weeks you'll slowly build up strength and endurance—never pushing yourself too far or too fast—until, by the tenth week, you'll join the 25 per cent or so of British adults who get at least 30 minutes of moderate-intensity physical activity three or more times a week.

A DIET THAT'S REALISTIC

Most programmes put all overweight women on the same 1000- to 1200-calorie diet. But one diet plan does *not* fit all. For many, a 1200-calorie diet is self-defeating because it cuts food intake too drastically. They try to comply, but hunger usually wins. The *Strong Women Stay Slim* programme has 1200-, 1600-, and 2000-calorie plans, so it adjusts for everyone. You'll learn how to **eat to the limit**—to adjust your intake so you continue to lose, while eating as much healthy food as possible.

Let's face it: if you're trying to lose weight, you can't eat as much as you want of whatever you want. But if deprivation has kept you from succeeding in the past, I can offer you two important promises:

- ◆ **First, you can eat the foods you love.** There are no forbidden foods on this programme. You can have a slice of chocolate cake on your birthday; you can order barbecued ribs at your favourite restaurant.

♦ **Second, you never need to be hungry.** In addition to ample meals and snacks, you can have almost unlimited amounts of certain filling and nutritious foods.

A VIBRANT NEW LIFESTYLE

Of course, you want to lose weight to improve your appearance. But I hope you're also concerned about your health. Some weight-reduction measures force you to choose between looking good and feeling good, but not this one. Instead of worrisome side effects, this programme offers added *benefits*—increased vitality and strength, improved mood and sleep, better balance and flexibility, plus reduced risk of heart disease, diabetes, cancer, arthritis, and other debilitating conditions.

♦　♦　♦

I'm not just happy about the weight loss; I'm happy about how I'm losing weight. I love being strong. I like knowing that my diet is healthy and that I'm getting regular aerobic exercise. My husband keeps telling me how proud he is of what I'm doing.
— Alexandra

♦　♦　♦

TEN WEEKS TO A NEW YOU

The *Strong Women Stay Slim* programme lets you bypass the dangers and deprivation of quick-weight-loss programmes. You lose weight steadily, at the sensible rate that doctors recommend—200 to 900 grams (7 to 32 oz) a week. But thanks to strength training, you'll see *results* just as quickly as with risky, counterproductive quick-loss programmes. As you trade fat for muscle (which is more compact), you'll look trimmer. You'll also see fast results in the form of increased energy and strength. Most women experience thrilling improvements in less than a month.

Here's where you'll be at the end of ten weeks:

- **If you needed to lose 2.5 to 4.5 kilos (5½ to 10 lb)**, you will have reached this goal by losing 0.25 to 0.5 kilo (½ to 1 lb) per week over the entire ten-week period. You may have been battling that same 2 or 5 kilos (4½ to 11 lb) for years! Now, thanks to weight loss and exercise, you should be shapelier as well as slimmer. And the weight is gone for good.

- **If you needed to lose between 5 and 20 kilos (11 and 44 lb)**, you will have lost about 4.5 kilos (10 lb). I realise that may not sound like much if you're used to the quick results of fad diets. But because you've also been doing strength training and aerobic exercise, you'll probably look much more than 4.5 kilos (10 lb) slimmer. More important, this time you won't have to put up with inconvenient (and unnecessary) food restrictions or go hungry. Instead, you'll be following a sensible plan that will let you lose the remaining weight and stay slim and healthy for the rest of your life.

- **If you need to lose more than 20 kilos (44 lb)**, you'll shed 5 to 10 kilos (11 to 22 lb) during the first ten weeks—a significant start. Adding to this loss will be the slimming effects of your fitness programme. For the first time you'll have a food plan that doesn't starve you, and exercise that allows you to succeed. I'm sure you'll be brimming with self-confidence. Just keep going, and your weight loss will continue. You're establishing the lifestyle that will keep the weight off forever.

You can expect other changes, regardless of where you started:

- You'll feel stronger and more capable physically; you'll have much more energy.

- You'll sleep better at night.

- Your chronic aches and pains may disappear.

♦ Your self-esteem will increase; you'll feel happier. You'll look
   in the mirror and like what you see.

Not visible but vitally important are the improvements to your
cardiovascular system, your muscles, your bones, and your balance.

♦ ♦ ♦

*In the past when I went on a diet, I would try to motivate myself
by thinking about reaching my ideal size. But the task seemed
overwhelming. Eventually I'd say to myself, "Forget it—I'll never
get there." This time I'm getting immediate gratification, and that
keeps me going. My strength and energy increased right away; my
stress level is way down. I'm out of bed before the alarm goes off.
And people are starting to comment on how much better I look.*
   —Ruth

♦ ♦ ♦

WHAT THIS BOOK PROVIDES

You're about to start a programme that will change how you live. You'll lose
weight safely and permanently. This book will tell you everything you
need to know. Here's what it gives you:

UP-TO-THE-MINUTE SCIENTIFIC INFORMATION

The more you know, the more motivated you will be.

♦ Chapter 2 explains what it takes to control appetite and
   get your metabolism on your side. You'll learn why some
   diets fail—and why this one will work.

♦ Chapter 3 explains exactly how strength training—along
   with a more active lifestyle—promotes weight loss,
   tightens and trims your figure, and offers significant

health benefits. Exercise not only helps you look and feel better right now, it also reduces your long-term risk for almost all major chronic diseases. No medication can match it.

◆ Chapter 4 explains how a healthy diet helps you live slimmer and longer. Good nutrition tames hunger and cravings, so you lose weight more easily and keep it off.

◆ DETAILED STEP-BY-STEP INSTRUCTIONS

The book gives you complete directions, and tells you how to adapt this programme to your particular needs.

◆ Chapter 7 gives you a strength-training programme—six basic moves designed for weight loss, plus optional supplementary exercises you can add later.

◆ Chapter 8 provides directions for becoming more active, with self-tests that ensure you get on the right track and progress safely.

◆ Chapter 9 presents the food plan, with basic instructions and menus that can be adapted to any lifestyle.

◆ Chapter 10 will help you put everything together, so you're on your way.

◆ Chapter 12 answers common questions about the programme.

◆ MOTIVATIONAL SAVVY

It's not easy to make changes in your life, even when you know they're important. In our research at Tufts, where we need to follow volunteers for many months, we've worked very hard to learn how to motivate participants. I'm very proud of the fact that our dropout rates are among the lowest reported in the medical literature. Even if you're not coming into our labs every week, what we've learned can work for you.

- Chapter 5 draws upon sports psychology to explain the mental secrets of successful weight loss.

- Chapter 6 helps you decide what you should weigh—the number may surprise you.

- Chapter 11 tells you how to keep yourself on track once you get started—including how to overcome any obstacles you may encounter.

◆ TWO WEEKS OF INNOVATIVE MENUS AND RECIPES BASED ON THE FOOD PLAN

To get you off to a good start, I asked cookbook author Steven Raichlen to prepare two weeks of menus and recipes. As the recipes came in, I had great fun trying them. You'll be delighted—as my family and I were—to see how well you can eat on this plan.

You are about to start a programme that will change your life forever. You're taking charge, and doing something wonderful for yourself. Expect a very positive experience, right from the start.

2

WHY DO
WOMEN GAIN
WEIGHT?

After my daughter was born, I couldn't lose weight. I started to think about diet pills, even though I knew that was a dangerous road. I tried a commercial diet organisation for a while, but it was expensive. Besides, I don't like to be told what I can and can't eat.
— *Therese*

♦ ♦ ♦

You're smart, you're disciplined about work—yet you can't seem to lose weight. Or maybe you're able to lose (you've done it dozens of times), but you can't keep the weight off. You know it's not just a matter of willpower, because you have plenty of this in other areas of your life. The situation is all the more frustrating because weight loss sounds simple: *Just eat less.* You've probably heard this well-meant advice from friends and relatives. You may even have told yourself the same thing. But you don't know why it's so difficult to do.

In fact, weight loss isn't simple at all. Intricate and powerful systems in our bodies regulate both appetite and metabolism in what seems like a conspiracy to keep us at our present weight. To make matters worse, stringent dieting actually exacerbates the situation by slowing metabolism and leaving the appetite unsatisfied. Fortunately, solutions are starting to emerge—and it's becoming increasingly clear that "Just eat less" is not the answer.

THE DELICATE BALANCE

My work gives me the opportunity to talk with women of all ages and sizes about their weight problems. Some have been heavy all their lives; others are trying to get rid of the excess from their last pregnancy, or they're worried about gaining during menopause. These women are very different from each other, but many of them tell me the same thing:

I can't seem to lose weight, but I really don't eat that much.

And I respond: *I know you're right!*

Usually they're very surprised—other people always assume they over-eat. But that's often not the problem.

Whether you gain or lose weight depends on your **energy balance**—how much food energy you burn compared with how much you consume. This energy is measured in **calories**.

Food energy—measured in calories—is what keeps our bodies alive and functioning. To maintain a consistent weight, our calorie intake must equal calorie output. If we eat more than we burn, the excess is stored as body fat. All of us have days when we go way over on intake, but the equation doesn't have to balance every single day so long as things generally come out even. I always feel bad when I hear a woman berating herself for enjoying good food at a party. Special events are rarely responsible for weight problems. Rather, the kilos accumulate because of *small but consistent* imbalances. Just 50 calories a day of extra intake or insufficient calorie expenditure adds up to 2.25 kilos (5 lb) a year. When a woman tells me that creeping weight gain has left her about 20 kilos (44 lb) heavier than she was ten years ago, I know that 150 calories a day could account for it. Those dramatic government statistics about the increasing prevalence of overweight in women, which I mentioned in Chapter 1, reflect very small imbalances, not rampant gluttony.

When you hear about a 250-calorie excess, you might automatically think of food—a woman could get 50 extra calories from half an apple or a few dry biscuits, or simply by adding cream and sugar to a cup of coffee. Until recently, experts also focused mostly on the intake side of the energy balance equation. But decades ago a different hypothesis was proposed by the late Dr Jean Mayer, the famous dietitian after whom our Tufts research centre is named. Dr Mayer believed that overweight usually was caused *not* by excessive calorie intake but by insufficient calorie expenditure—the other side of the equation. When he first proposed this idea, back in the 1950s, most dietitians thought he was way off target. Since then, accumulated evidence has proven that he was absolutely right:

The surprising reason why women gain weight is that they're burning too few calories.

We now know that most women are getting heavier not because they eat more. Moreover, it doesn't take much of a discrepancy to cause significant weight gain over time. But the balance can just as easily be tipped in the other direction. Weight loss doesn't require stringent dieting or gruelling exercise. Small but consistent changes can produce a remarkable difference—and strength training makes it easy.

IS YOUR METABOLISM WORKING AGAINST YOU?

My husband eats whatever he wants—fried chicken, full-cream ice cream, you name it—and he can still fit into trousers he bought twenty years ago. How come I gain weight if I so much as look at a crisp? It's not fair!
— *Alexandra*

◆　◆　◆

I get questions like this all the time. So many women look around and are baffled to see other people eating more but weighing less. They wonder whether there's something wrong with them. Could it be their genes, or maybe a thyroid problem? Is it just an inevitable consequence of being a woman or of getting older? Yes, all of these factors can play a role, and they help explain why weight loss is so difficult.

The calories we burn fall into three categories:

- **Basal metabolism**—the energy our body needs to remain alive—accounts for 50 to 75 per cent of our daily energy/calorie expenditure.

- **Digestion**—we use about 10 per cent of the calories we consume to process food.

- **Physical activity**—15 to 40 per cent of our calorie expenditure is used for activities above the basal metabolic baseline.

As you'll see, nature may indeed be working against you. Even so, there's a great deal you can do to rev up your metabolism.

BASAL METABOLISM

Your resting metabolic rate (RMR), or basal metabolism, is the energy you consume when you're awake but not using any calories to move. In the laboratory we measure RMR first thing in the morning, before our volunteers get out of bed. Basal metabolism reflects all the work your body does to sustain life: the beating of your heart, the activities of all your other organs, the functioning of your brain, temperature regulation, and the tiny repairs that keep your muscles and bones in working order.

Metabolism, as Alexandra says, is not fair. Your genetic heritage helps determine your metabolic rate, as well as the shape of your body. However, the lifestyle you picked up from your parents contributes too—and that part can be altered. Men really do have an advantage, as I'll explain. It's also true that our basal metabolic rate typically decreases as we get older. But as you'll see, behind the sex and age differences are differences in body composition and activity. Indeed, the single most important factor in determining RMR is the amount of lean tissue in our body. This is very good news because it means **we can increase our basal metabolic rate by 15 per cent or more, simply by building muscle and becoming more active.**

Why It's Easier For Men

A woman of average weight has a resting metabolic rate of about 1300 calories; but the average normal-weight man has an RMR of about 1650 calories—a 350 calorie advantage! Hormones explain some of it, but not much.

HOW TO ESTIMATE YOUR
BASAL METABOLIC RATE

Precise measurement of the basal metabolic rate requires elaborate scientific equipment. However, you can use the following equation, called the Harris-Benedict formula, to make an estimate. This version is calibrated for women; although it takes weight, height and age into account, other factors—especially the amount of lean tissue in your body—are also very important. You will need a calculator.

4.4 × [weight in pounds] + 4.7 × [height in inches] − 4.7 [age in years] + 655.

Here's how to do the calculation:

Step 1: Multiply your weight in pounds by 4.4 _____

Step 2: Multiply your height in inches by 4.7 _____

Step 3: Add answers from Step 1 and Step 2 _____

Step 4: Multiply your age in years by 4.7 _____

Step 5: Subtract Step 4 answer from Step 3 _____

Step 6: Add 655 to the answer from Step 5 _____

If your weight is normal or slightly above normal, the answer in Step 6 is a good approximation of your BMR—the number of calories you burn each day simply by being alive. If you're very overweight, this will slightly overestimate your BMR by 10 to 15 per cent.

Example: Linda weighs 173 pounds; she's 5 feet 5 inches tall, and 38 years old.

Step 1: Multiply your weight in pounds by 4.4 _____761_____

Step 2: Multiply your height in inches by 4.7 _____306_____

Step 3: Add answers from Step 1 and Step 2 _____1067_____

Step 4: Multiply your age in years by 4.7 _____179_____

Step 5: Subtract Step 4 answer from Step 3 _____888_____

Step 6: Add 2741 to the answer from Step 5 _____1543_____

Linda's BMR is 1,543 calories.

Far more important is the difference in men's body composition. He weighs 73 kilos (160 lb); she weighs 57 (125 lb). He's leaner as well as heavier, with 12 per cent body fat to her 20 per cent. So his metabolism is driven by 64 kilos (140 lb) of lean tissue, compared with just 46 kilos (101 lb) for her.

In other words, it's not his testosterone, it's his muscles.

What Happens As We Get Older

If you haven't yet experienced this change for yourself, you've probably heard your older women friends and relatives complain about it:

I'm not eating any differently, but I'm gaining weight.
I can't have dessert any more.

The explanation is very simple: as we age, we usually burn fewer calories. The resting metabolic rate of an average 60 year old is about 200 calories a day lower than the RMR of a typical 30 year old. Most of the difference can be explained by body composition. Starting around age 40, most women lose about 15 grams (½ oz) of muscle each year (and gain at least that much body fat); they also lose smaller amounts of bone. These changes accelerate at perimenopause and during early menopause. At this time of her life, a woman can lose 2.5 kilograms (5½ lb) of muscle in just five years— unless she compensates with strengthening exercise.

Physical Activity Kick-starts The Engine

We've known for a long time that exercise can compensate for the age-related decline in basal metabolism. Intriguing new research suggests that physical activity does even more: it can actually halt this change.

Investigators at the University of Colorado compared sedentary and active postmenopausal women aged 50 to 72 with women aged 21 to 35. The older women who were sedentary showed the expected decrease in RMR compared with their younger counterparts. But *older women who were physically active had the same RMRs on average as active women half their age!*

Overly Stringent Dieting Undermines Metabolism

Our bodies seem to think we're still living as hunter-gatherers when drought might strike or the hunting might be bad, instead of around the corner from a supermarket. When a woman cuts calories too drastically, her body has no idea she's trying to lose weight—so her thyroid gland leaps into action to protect her from starvation.

The thyroid gland, a small butterfly-shaped organ located in the neck, regulates metabolism by secreting a hormone called thyroxine. The amount of thyroxine you secrete is influenced by what you eat. If you consume fewer calories than your body burns, your thyroid tries to compensate by cutting back on thyroxine: your metabolism slows down and you feel sluggish, so you don't move around as much. These are *not* abnormalities—your thyroid is just doing its job and trying to conserve body tissue. Usually the effect is too small to be noticed. However, it becomes significant if a woman fasts or follows a very low-calorie diet. Such extremes can cause her RMR to plummet by as much as 30 per cent. That's why it's so important to eat enough when you're trying to lose weight.

This perfectly normal thyroid response should not be confused with thyroid disorders that affect weight. Some women gain because their thyroid glands are under-active, a condition called **hypothyroidism**. Symptoms include not only sluggish metabolism, but also fatigue, depression, dry skin, constipation, and sensitivity to cold. Though hypothyroidism is uncommon, even in overweight women, anyone who suspects she might have this problem can take a simple blood test to find out for sure. The condition is readily treated with synthetic thyroid hormone.

FOOD HELPS YOU BURN CALORIES

It takes calories to burn calories. About 10 per cent of your daily calorie intake is used to process that food. In other words, if you consume about 2000 calories a day, approximately 200 calories are burned just for digestion. Though this is an important part of the energy balance equation, you can't do much to change it. *There's no scientific evidence that particular combinations of foods will help you burn more calories.* Some foods—including high-fibre grains, protein foods, fruits, and vegetables—do require extra calories to digest. However, the difference is insignificant.

THE SIMPLEST WAY TO USE EXTRA CALORIES: PHYSICAL ACTIVITY

Physical activity is the part of calorie expenditure that varies the most from person to person, and it's also the easiest to modify. Any woman can significantly increase the number of calories she burns through activity.

Remember, it doesn't take much: I've already explained that for many women, the difference between slim and heavy is as little as 50 calories a day. Also, I'm not just talking about those activities we think of as exercise, like jogging around a track or taking a step-aerobics class. *All* physical activity counts.

Let me use myself as an example. I have a hearty appetite and eat about 2200 calories a day, yet I never gain weight. There's nothing magical about my metabolism. In fact, because I'm petite, my resting metabolic rate is slightly lower than average—only about 1285 calories a day. My body uses another 10 per cent of my intake, around 215 calories a day, for digestion.

What about the remaining 700 calories? If I were sedentary, I'd burn only about 285 extra calories a day; unless I cut way back on food, I'd gain weight. But because I'm physically active, I use up the entire 700 calories and my weight remains the same.

As I'll explain in Chapter 8, I strength train twice a week; I also make a point of getting at least 45 minutes of aerobic exercise three or more times a week. That might sound like a lot of exercise, but if you add it all up, it averages out to only about 100 calories per day. What keeps my weight stable is all the rest of my physical activity: walking whenever possible instead of taking the car or bus; moving around the room when I talk on the phone instead of sitting in a chair; playing active games with my children.

Modern conveniences have pushed physical activity out of our lives. We put telephone extensions all over the house so we don't need to walk from room to room; we toss laundry into the washing machine instead of labouring over a sink; we cut the grass with a motor mower instead of the human-powered kind. These are trivial changes, but they add up. In fact, they may explain most of the collective weight gain Britons have experienced over the past several decades. Believe me, I'm not suggesting you return to the scrub board! But the more active you become, the higher your metabolism will be.

Because overweight makes moving harder, women often pick up sedentary habits along with extra kilos: they use the remote control instead of getting up to change channels; they ask a child to fetch the mail. These patterns can be subtle. One fascinating study, done long ago by Dr Jean Mayer and colleagues, filmed heavy and normal girls as they played tennis, then analysed their moves. You'd think that all the players would be equally active, but they weren't. The normal-weight youngsters were in constant motion during the game, but their overweight counterparts hardly budged except when hitting the ball.

When women become stronger, they naturally become more active. At the end of a year of strength training, the women in my *JAMA* study were an astonishing 27 per cent more active, despite having been asked not to begin additional exercise. When you begin strength training, you'll experience the same vitalising change. I hope you'll also make a conscious effort to build more physical activity into your daily life—I'll give you lots of specific suggestions in Chapter 8. Here's a special incentive: the more you weigh, the more calories you'll burn when you get active. For instance, a 53-kilogram (117-lb) woman might use up about 50 calories during a brisk ten-minute walk. But a 90-kilogram (198-lb) woman who took exactly the same walk would burn about 75 calories—it takes extra energy to move more weight.

FAT ISN'T ALL BAD!

Our bodies are *supposed* to contain some fat. Here's what it does for us:

- **Provides an energy reserve**—Our fat stores are nature's way of enabling us to withstand starvation.

- **Cushions our bodies**—Vital organs, like the kidney, liver, and intestines, are padded with a protective layer of fat.

- **Acts as insulation**—The layer of fat just under your skin helps keep you warm in the winter. (Of course, if you have too much fat, you'll get overheated in the summer.)

- **Synthesises oestrogen**—Extra fat reduces hot flushes and other symptoms of menopause (but unfortunately also increases the risk of breast cancer).

◆ ◆ ◆

I live in a two-storey house with a basement, and I used to avoid going up and down the steps—this was very efficient, but not very smart since I want to use up more calories. A couple of weeks ago

I decided to give myself points for climbing stairs. I put an index card and pencil at the top of the stairs, and every time I come upstairs, I get a point. It has worked! When I started, I made five to ten trips a day; now I'm up to 15 to 20.
— *Jayne*

♦ ♦ ♦

HOW WOMEN GET HIT WITH A DOUBLE WHAMMY

Once you understand the importance of basal metabolism and physical activity in the energy balance equation, you can see why women are so vulnerable to weight problems at key times in their lives.

Postpartum Plumpness

I'd always been slender, but things changed when I became pregnant. During the first few months I felt nauseated and tired, and I discovered that sugar gave me relief. That's when I began using food for comfort. Also, my lifestyle became more sedentary, especially after my second child was born. One day I woke up and realised that I weighed exactly what I'd weighed when I delivered my first baby—except I wasn't pregnant.
— *Martha*

♦ ♦ ♦

An 11- to 16-kilogram (23- to 35-lb) weight gain is healthy during pregnancy. Extra fluid and the developing baby account for most of that; your body also accumulates fat reserves. After birth, some women quickly return to their usual weight. But for others, the extra pounds linger. Though the problem has a physical origin, it's often compounded by all the changes motherhood brings.

Life with a new baby is hectic, but most women become more sedentary in the postpartum months. At the same time that they're burning fewer calories through physical activity, other factors conspire to make them eat more: often they're not getting enough sleep, and research suggests that fatigue is easily confused with hunger. They're at home, where food is more readily available, and their usual meal patterns are disrupted. On top of everything else, new mothers often experience the mild form of depression known as the "baby blues," which can lead to the kind of "comfort eating" Martha describes. As the kilos mount up, unhappiness increases and the problem gets worse.

MONTHLY WEIGHT FLUCTUATIONS

Though we experience premenstrual changes regularly, it's hard not to be dismayed by them—the weight gain, the bloated feeling, and often the voracious appetite. These problems are real, but fortunately only temporary. During the week to ten days before menstruation, women retain extra water and therefore put on a kilo or two (2 to 4½ lb). But they lose both liquid and weight by the time their period ends. Increased hunger does make many women eat more when they're premenstrual. However, there's a corresponding rise in metabolic rate that usually compensates for it.

Women who take birth control pills—which mimic the second half of the menstrual cycle—often experience mild versions of the same changes. Usually their body adapts in a month or two and the symptoms disappear. If you take oral contraceptives and have persistent weight problems, talk to your doctor. The solution could be as simple as a change to another pill formulation.

Menopausal Metamorphosis

I'm a breast cancer survivor. Chemotherapy made me go into menopause, and I started to gain weight. Four kilos (9 lb) hit me like a ton of bricks. Then another four crept on—in no time I weighed 75 kilos (165 lb), more than I'd ever been in my life. I didn't feel well: my lower back hurt all the time; I didn't have a lot of energy. I tried skipping meals and starving myself, but I continued to gain.

— Nancy

♦ ♦ ♦

I've already explained that women lose muscle when they start menopause. We know that hormonal changes are a contributing factor, but some of the loss is caused by decreased activity. Here too, a vicious circle begins: as women lose muscle, activity becomes more difficult. This leads to weight gain, which makes physical activity even harder. Meanwhile, lowered self-esteem and depression enter the picture, and may result in excess eating.

IS YOUR APPETITE OUT OF CONTROL?

Our appetite for food—like our instinctive need to breathe, drink, or sleep—is one of the biological mechanisms that keep us alive. But many women describe their hunger as an unreasonable and powerful force:

> Half an hour after a big meal, I'm ravenous all over again.
> Once I start, I can't stop—it's like a truck rolling downhill with no brakes.
> When cravings hit, I can't think about anything else.

The command centre for our appetite is in a part of the brain called the **hypothalamus**. When we need food, the hypothalamus sends out signals that we're hungry. After we've eaten, the message changes and the hypothalamus announces that we're satiated. We don't yet fully understand all the processes involved, but we know that healthy eating and physical activity can help tame an unruly appetite.

Because hunger and satiety are so important to our well-being, nature has multiple mechanisms to deliver information to the hypothalamus.

Stomach Contractions

Our stomach contracts when it has been empty for a while, producing that tight feeling we call "hunger pangs". After we've eaten and our stomach is distended by food, we sense that we're full. This is the first signal of satiation, and it's one we can enhance with savvy food choices. If we drink plenty of fluids and select high-bulk but low-calorie foods (such as fibre-rich vegetables and whole grains), we'll feel full more quickly.

BLOOD SUGAR

During digestion, food is broken down into sugar, which enters the bloodstream for distribution to our cells. The hypothalamus monitors the amount of sugar in our blood. As the level goes up, the hypothalamus senses that we've eaten. Later, depletion of blood sugar signals that we need to eat again.

Nature probably intended us to consume small quantities of food throughout the day rather than getting most of our calories in just three meals. Our bodies don't always cope very well with the resulting "sugar spikes." Sometimes blood sugar levels shoot too high and then fall too rapidly, causing us to feel hungry when we've really had enough.

Wise food choices can help reduce these fluctuations in blood sugar, as I'll explain in Chapter 4. If your diet is high in complex carbohydrates, such as vegetables and whole grains, sugar is released more gradually and you feel full longer. Being strong and active also helps: the muscles act as a storage buffer for sugar, which means that levels in the blood are more consistent.

SIGNALS FROM THE INTESTINES

When food leaves the stomach and enters the small intestines, the intestinal lining releases several hormones. We know from experiments in animals that these hormones are powerful appetite suppressants. One of them, called **cholecystokinin** (CCK), also seems to contribute to the calming effect we experience after eating. CCK is especially responsive to fat in the diet.

It's useful to remember that some satiety signals are not triggered until food is well along in the digestive process. That's one reason that it's so important to eat slowly, and to give your body a chance to realise it's been fed. Otherwise you may unwittingly overeat, then feel uncomfortably full later.

SEROTONIN AND OTHER CHEMICALS IN THE BRAIN

After we eat—particularly when we have foods rich in carbohydrates or dairy proteins—the brain releases chemicals, called neurotransmitters, that act on the nervous system. The best known of these neurotransmitters is **serotonin**, which not only influences hunger and satiety but also has a soothing effect. Many anti-depressant and anti-anxiety medications work by increasing serotonin levels or by making the brain more sensitive to existing supplies. If you reach for carbohydrate-rich food when you feel tense or unhappy, you're actually medicating yourself. Serotonin is very important, but it's just one of more than 500 neurotransmitters in the brain. Quite likely, others affect mood and appetite too. I expect we'll hear more about them as research continues.

Physical activity triggers the release of mood-affecting chemicals too. These hormones, called endorphins, are believed to be responsible for the anti-depression and calming effect of exercise. Endorphins also may help account for the fact that hunger seems to be diminished for two to three hours

THE DEPRESSED-SLUGGISH-HUNGRY SYNDROME

I vividly remember the autumn when I gained 9 kilos (20 lb). I was depressed. I drank too much red wine with too much dinner every night, and spent a lot of time after my son went to bed lying on the couch eating my way through big bags of mini chocolate bars.
— Jill

◆ ◆ ◆

Nearly every woman I know has sunk into this spiral at some time in her life. She feels unhappy and lethargic; she turns to food for comfort and for energy. So she gains weight—and then she feels even worse.

Each of these problems could be addressed individually. She could see a therapist for the depression, lethargy, and low self-esteem; improved nutrition could help her lose weight. But the most effective way to break out of this syndrome is with physical activity. Exercise lifts depression, combats lethargy, and makes weight loss easier. Strengthening exercise is especially helpful, because a woman sees significant changes in just a few weeks.

following vigorous exercise. Another contributor could be the slight elevation in body temperature with exercise, similar to the appetite-depressing effects of fever. Though more research is needed to settle the matter, many women have told me that taking a brisk walk helps them tame between-meal hunger—and this is one appetite suppressant I don't hesitate to recommend.

SIGNALS FROM OUR FAT CELLS

You may have heard of the fat cell theory of excess weight—the idea that people reach adulthood with a certain number of fat cells, and that these cells demand to be refilled if they become depleted. There's some truth to this. Our fat cells produce a protein called **leptin** that plays an important role in appetite regulation.

When leptin reaches the hypothalamus, it triggers a receptor that puts the brakes on production of a neurotransmitter called **neuropeptide Y (NPY)**. NPY is not only the brain's most potent appetite stimulant, but also a powerful metabolic suppressant. If we lose a little fat, we produce a little less leptin and have a corresponding increase in NPY. In other words, if you eat less on one day, you feel hungrier the next day and eat more.

Many scientists believe that this interaction between leptin and NPY may be responsible for the **set point** for weight—a weight that our body seems to return to, no matter how hard we try to lose. I prefer to use the term **settling point**, because there's evidence that this point is subject to change. One mechanism seems to be physical activity. We know that physical activity creates biochemical changes in the brain—that's why exercise relieves anxiety and depression. Some of these changes appear to affect NPY, which may explain the appetite-suppressing effects of physical activity. Though this hasn't yet been confirmed by research, I suspect we'll eventually have solid evidence that increasing physical activity can actually reset your "normal" weight.

IS LEPTIN THE ANSWER?

About forty years ago, scientists conducted an experiment in which they surgically connected the blood systems of pairs of mice, one normal and one (called the OB/OB mouse) that had been genetically altered to be overweight. OB/OB mice usually spend their days eating and sleeping; they gain weight rapidly and develop a characteristic round shape. But when these roly-poly mice were connected to normal mice, they suddenly changed their ways. Their metabolic rate increased and they ate less, became much more active and lost weight. Obviously there was something magical in the blood of the normal mice.

In 1994 Jeffrey Friedman, Ph.D., and his colleagues at Rockefeller University finally identified the remarkable substance: leptin. When bred-to-be-fat OB/OB mice are given leptin, they become slim. Excited by such promising results, a drug company paid US$20 million for the commercial rights to leptin. Human studies are under way to see whether administering leptin—or making the hypothalamus more sensitive to it—could prevent the surge in NPY that produces raging appetite and sluggish metabolism.

Though this is a very promising area of research, remember that the body has other independent mechanisms that regulate appetite and metabolism. Defects in these systems may account for excess weight in some people. If leptin turns out to be the answer, individuals who benefit from leptin treatment probably will have to continue taking it, much as diabetics require insulin.

THE THREE WEIGHT-LOSS STRATEGIES THAT REALLY WORK

If you've ever tried to lose weight, you know it isn't easy. A recent Harris poll reported that women dieters had attempted to lose weight an average of 14 times! According to a survey by *Prevention* magazine, 70 per cent of women who go on a diet hit a plateau before they reach their goal. Discouraged, nearly all of them give up and return to their previous eating habits.

Yes, weight loss is difficult—as I've just explained, your metabolic system and appetite seem determined to thwart your efforts. But we're learning that, with the right approach, you can break through. New findings on the benefits of strength training are enormously encouraging. Another source of helpful new insights is the National Weight Control Registry, an exciting project at the University of Pittsburgh. Investigators have located hundreds of men and women who have been able to take off significant amounts of weight and keep it off. They've just published the first in what I hope will be a series of reports about their volunteers—629 women and 155 men who have lost an average of 30 kilograms (66 lb), and have maintained at least 13.5 kilograms (30 lb) of that loss for an average of 5.5 years.

The latest research indicates that three strategies are the key to successful long-term weight loss.

#1: BUILD LEAN TISSUE BY STRENGTH TRAINING

The more muscle you have, the more calories you burn. This important change comes partly from a revved-up metabolism and partly from increased physical activity—an automatic consequence of greater strength. Strengthening exercise also protects your muscle and bone, so you don't lose precious lean tissue along with fat.

#2: GET MOVING!

Experts now agree that most people are overweight not because they eat too much but because they exercise too little. Vigorous aerobic exercise—the kind that makes you breathe harder—is just part of what's needed. Even more important is increasing your activity throughout the day. The more energetically you move, the more calories you will use. The crucial importance of exercise for maintaining weight loss is underscored by the experience of the successful dieters in the National Weight Control Registry: an astonishing 89 per cent of them were physically active.

#3: FLY JUST BELOW YOUR BODY'S HUNGER RADAR

Cutting calories is usually necessary. However, most women can lose weight successfully on a wholesome, well-balanced diet that supplies 1600 to 2000 calories per day—provided they're physically active. If you try to speed weight loss by cutting calories more drastically, you might lose an extra kilogram or two for a couple of weeks. But restrictive, quick-loss diets are doomed by catastrophic metabolic drops. In the long run, you'll lose more weight—and keep it off more easily—if you eat more. A generous food plan is not only more enjoyable and more satisfying, it also provides more nutrients and thereby reduces hunger and cravings.

The *Strong Women Stay Slim* programme is designed to help you do all this. Perhaps the best part of the programme is that you don't have to compromise your health to take advantage of these weight-loss strategies. Indeed, as you'll see in Chapters 3 and 4, the same changes that will make you slim will have many other wonderful benefits.

HOW EXERCISE

TRANSFORMS YOUR BODY

I knew exercise was really important, but I was having a lot of trouble getting into it. I had a project at work that kept me sedentary; I had two little children at home—and I wasn't happy with myself. When I started strength training, everything became easier. After my legs got stronger, I began using a stationary bike. Then I added sit-ups. In a couple of months I lost 4.5 kilos (10 lb)
    — Martha

◆ ◆ ◆

Sometimes, after I've given a lecture that describes the remarkable benefits of physical activity, a woman will come up to me and say:

I'll start exercising after I lose weight.

If I ask her why she doesn't want to begin straightaway, she says:

What's the point in trying to get fit if I'm overweight? And besides, there's no way I'm going to a gym, riding my bike, or getting into a bathing suit when I look like this.

Ironically, the heavier a woman is, the more she will benefit from exercise. As I explained in Chapter 2, physical activity is the key to lasting weight loss. But that's not all. Exercise breaks through the sluggishness and depression that keep a woman stuck in unhealthy patterns she desperately wants to change. Getting active—even before she loses weight—gives her a new sparkle that makes her look and feel more attractive. The change goes deeper. Scientists now suspect that many of the medical problems blamed on excess weight are actually caused in large part by inactivity.

AN EPIDEMIC OF WEAKNESS

Behind the epidemic of excess weight in the United States is another epidemic that has received very little attention: the weakening of American women. (Generally speaking, this also applies to women throughout the western world.) A recent US study of 10,000 women aged 40 to 55 found that more than a quarter of them were so weak that they had difficulty with everyday activities—climbing a flight of stairs, carrying groceries or walking around the block. The heavier the woman, the more likely she was to experience disabling weakness.

What's happening to our strength? I've already explained that many women lose muscle when they diet. An inactive lifestyle also plays a role—"Use it or lose it" definitely applies to muscles. Even more pervasive is the shift in body composition that begins in mid-life. Starting around the age of 40, we typically lose muscle mass at the rate of about 160 grams (6 oz) a year, and we gain that much body fat or more. If nothing is done to prevent it, by the age of 80 we'll have only a third of the muscle we had at age 40. This change, called *sarcopenia* (from the Greek "sarco" for muscle or flesh and "penia" for loss) is one of the chief reasons for frailty and loss of vitality later in life.

The spiral of weakness and inactivity—which leads to further muscle loss and weakness—also explains why so many women put on weight as they get older. With less muscle they burn fewer calories, so it becomes easier and easier to gain. But when women start strength training, changes move in the other direction.

STARTING OFF STRONG

I hated the idea of exercise, but strength training sounded tolerable: I wouldn't have to wear special clothes, get down on the floor, move rapidly, or sweat. So I started lifting weights, and— surprise!—I was good at it. This got me interested in trying other exercise for the first time in my life.
— *Sarah*

◆ ◆ ◆

Strengthening exercise prepares your body for a more active lifestyle. A big part is that you're getting stronger, but there's more: strength training also improves your balance and flexibility, reducing your risk of injury.

GAINS IN STRENGTH, NOT BULK

Strength training enlarges muscle cells, enabling them to exert more force. When women hear this, they often worry that strength training will give them a bulky body-builder look. However, that doesn't happen on the *Strong Women Stay Slim* programme. Female (and for that matter, male) body builders follow a very different regimen. They lift much heavier weights and have lengthier workouts; some also take steroids and follow rigorous diets. The women in my studies don't go to these extremes. They become a lot stronger, but they usually wind up *smaller*, not larger. For example, in my *JAMA* osteoporosis study, volunteers gained only about 1.3 kilograms (3 lb) of muscle, but that was enough to make an enormous difference in their strength. At the same time, they lost 1.3 kilograms (3 lb) of fat. Since a kilo of fat takes up more room than a kilo of muscle, they became trimmer, not bulkier.

Increased strength isn't just a matter of bigger muscles. Two other changes are also important:

- **Nerve reactivation**—Muscles move when signals flash from the brain via nerves, telling muscle fibres to contract. Strength is lost not only because muscles shrink if they're inactive, but also because muscle-stimulating nerves become dormant. Strength training reactivates these nerves almost immediately, bringing more muscle cells into play. That's why you'll see big results quickly, without much change in muscle size.

◆ **Enzyme enhancements**—As strength training stimulates your muscles, certain beneficial enzymes increase, improving your body's ability to process oxygen and fuel. This change also contributes to strength.

◆   ◆   ◆

I have been strength training for about ten weeks, and it amazes me how quickly my body has responded. I'd been walking on a treadmill for 30 minutes, three times a week, for approximately a year. I had been stuck at the same speed for several months, not due to cardiovascular difficulty but because my legs would get too fatigued. Since starting strength training, I have increased my speed twice and am not having any problems with my legs. I'm thrilled!

— Denise

◆   ◆   ◆

BETTER BALANCE

Our balancing ability starts to decline in mid-life. This change happens so slowly that most of us don't notice it until we're in our seventies. Strength training helps to halt the deterioration and turn it around. In my *JAMA* osteoporosis study, the women who didn't exercise scored 8.5 per cent lower on a balance test after just one year. In contrast, the volunteers who strength trained showed a dramatic improvement: their balance test scores increased by 14 per cent.

We know that older women are very much aware of impaired balance, and many curtail their physical activity to avoid falling. Younger women also may become less active in response to subtle changes in their balance, even if they don't fully realise why. Regardless of your age, improved balance will certainly reduce your risk of falls and injury—and may also boost your physical self-confidence.

IMPROVED FLEXIBILITY

When your joints are flexible, sports and other physical activities become much easier. Although flexibility has not been the main focus of my research, many of my volunteers are delighted to find that their shoulders, knees, and ankles become much more flexible as a result of strength training.

◆ ◆ ◆

Last year, if I sat on the floor with my legs straight in front of me and I bent forward, I could barely reach 10 centimetres (4 inches) beyond my knees. Now, after eight months of strength training, I can stretch 70 centimetres (27 inches) further and almost touch my toes.
        —Judith

◆ ◆ ◆

EXERCISE EXTENDS AND IMPROVES YOUR LIFE

If doctors could prescribe exercise in pill form, it would be the single most widely prescribed drug in the world.
        —Dr Robert Butler

◆ ◆ ◆

Dr Butler is one of my favourite mentors, and this is my favourite quote about exercise. Strength training has powerful health benefits by itself. You gain even more because your new strength encourages you to become more active.

When I was a graduate student in the early 1980s, we were just beginning to realise that physical activity could reduce the risk of cardiovascular disease. Back then we also knew that being active was important for weight control. It's been exciting to watch the list of benefits expand every year. Accumulated evidence was so extensive by 1996 that the Surgeon General of the United States, in collaboration with the Centers for Disease Control and Prevention, issued a special report on physical activity that concluded:

Moderate exercise is just as essential to a healthy life as good nutrition, seat belts, and avoiding cigarettes.

People who exercise regularly not only live longer, they live *better*. They're healthier and have fewer disabilities; they're happier and more productive—and they look better too. What's more, all these gains come with few, if any, negative consequences.

Perfect Partners

Strengthening exercise is enormously valuable—but it doesn't train your heart and lungs. For that you need **aerobic exercise**. An aerobic activity is one that causes your heart to beat faster and your breathing rate to increase. This happens during the exercise because your muscles are working and calling for more fuel and oxygen.

Aerobic exercise is the perfect complement to strength training, especially if you want to lose weight. Here's what it does additionally:

- Burns calories, which contributes to weight loss and loss of fat generally.

- Helps burn fat in your abdominal area.

- Aids in toning your muscles.

- Tames your appetite, bringing it in line with your energy expenditure.

- Provides an emotional lift.

- Improves the health of your cardiovascular system and lungs.

Being Fit Helps Even If You're Overweight

Much of what we know about the relationship between lifestyle and health comes from ambitious research projects that follow thousands of people over many years. Steven Blair, P.E.D., and his colleagues at the Cooper Institute for Aerobics Research in Dallas, Texas, have done the largest such study focusing on exercise. Since 1970 they've recruited over 25,000 men and more than 7,000 women aged 20 to 88, all of whom agreed to be followed for seven to eight

THE #1 QUESTION WOMEN ASK ABOUT EXERCISE

I recently gave a talk about strength training at a retirement community, and afterwards I asked if anyone had questions. An attractive elderly woman immediately raised her hand. "I'm 88 years old," she said. "What can I do to firm up my abdomen?" I hear this question all the time, from all ages—adolescents up.

Here's how strength training and aerobic exercise deliver a one–two punch to firm and flatten your abdominal area:

◆ Strengthening exercise tones the muscles in your abdomen and back. It's easy to understand why the abdominal muscles are important, but how do the back muscles affect your appearance in front? Strong back muscles contribute to good posture, which makes your abdomen look flatter. Women who have poor posture from osteoporosis look thicker around the middle even if they don't gain weight.

◆ Aerobic exercise not only burns calories but specifically targets the layer of fat in the abdominal area, which is bad for health as well as appearance. In addition, certain aerobic activities—including walking, cycling, stair climbing, and cross-country skiing—help firm the abdominal and back muscles.

years. These volunteers underwent extensive physical examinations—including a treadmill test to assess fitness—and provided detailed personal information. The researchers know the volunteers' height and weight, their blood pressure and cholesterol profiles, their smoking habits, and their medical histories.

In 1996 Dr Blair and his associates wrote a fascinating report focused on those participants—601 men and 89 women—who died during their follow-up period. What was the biggest difference between the volunteers who died and the ones who survived? Not fat, but fitness. When other risk factors were held constant, those in the lowest fitness category had double the mortality rate of those whose fitness was medium or high. The findings were startling: fitness trumped all other risk factors, including excess weight, diabetes, elevated blood pressure, and high cholesterol. Only smoking came close.

People who were fat and fit had the same mortality risk as people who were lean and fit—and *much lower* mortality rates than those who were lean but unfit. Other research has confirmed these findings. **Being fit helps you live longer—no matter how much you weigh.**

EXERCISE TURNS BACK THE CLOCK

My mother lives in a retirement home. When I visit her I see women in their eighties and nineties, who never were encouraged to do anything physical—and now their lives are so impaired by their disabilities. That's prompted me to take active steps.
—Judith

♦ ♦ ♦

As you can see, physical activity has extraordinary rejuvenating effects. I'm not just talking about feeling more youthful, though of course that's one result. Exercise actually alters the body in ways that reverse or compensate for age-related declines.

After a year of strength training, the postmenopausal women in my *JAMA* study showed remarkable changes. Without taking drugs, they regained bone instead of losing it as women normally do at that age. They became stronger—in most cases stronger than they'd ever been in their lives. Their balance and flexibility improved. Because movement was so much easier, they spontaneously became more physically active. When we took stock of all these changes, we realised that *after just one year of strength training their bodies had become fifteen to twenty years more youthful.*

Aerobic exercise revitalises your cardiovascular system. Typically we lose cardiovascular fitness as we get older, especially if we're not active. One reason is that after age 40, our hearts gradually lose the ability to beat rapidly, so our maximum heart rate begins to decline. This change occurs even in those who remain physically fit, which helps explain why the performance of top athletes usually peaks when they're in their twenties and thirties. But few of us challenge our hearts to perform anywhere near their maximums. Far more significant for most women are the changes that result from inactivity—but these can be largely reversed by aerobic exercise. A study I did in the mid-1980s found that physically active women aged 50 to 70 had the same level of cardiovascular fitness as sedentary women half their age.

EXERCISE FIGHTS DISEASE AND DISABILITY

Physical activity makes a major contribution to health simply by helping women lose weight and keep it off. But the benefits go further. In addition, physical activity reduces the risk for many diseases; it may also counter symptoms if you already have a medical condition. Here's an up-to-the-minute summary—but I can promise that, as additional research is completed, there will be even more.

Cardiovascular Disease

Cardiovascular disease—heart disease and stroke—is the number one killer of both women and men. Overweight people have triple the normal risk. The best way to combat the danger is by a combination of weight loss, improved diet, and physical activity. But exercise is beneficial all by itself: it reduces blood pressure, decreases the level of harmful cholesterol in the blood, and improves the condition of blood vessels. These changes greatly reduce the risk of heart attacks and stroke.

Aerobic exercise conditions your cardiovascular system in three ways. It:

- increases the amount of blood you can pump with each heartbeat, which compensates for age-related limitations

- improves circulation by making your blood vessels healthier

- increases production of enzymes responsible for oxygen metabolism, allowing you to use oxygen more effectively.

What does this mean in real life? When your cardiovascular fitness improves, you have more energy; you don't find yourself gasping for breath if you have to move quickly. Activities that stopped being enjoyable because they were such a struggle become fun again.

Diabetes

An estimated 1.4 million Britons have diabetes. The disease, which interferes with sugar metabolism, kills more than 150,000 people a year in the

US and is one of the largest contributors to heart disease. Excess weight is strongly associated with adult-onset diabetes, by far the more prevalent form. By countering obesity, exercise works indirectly to reduce the risk of diabetes. In addition, physical activity contributes to metabolic changes that allow the body to process sugar more efficiently.

Cancer

Women are often surprised to hear that exercise can actually decrease their cancer risk, but studies of large groups of people show there really is a connection—especially with breast and colon cancer. What's the link? In the case of breast cancer, the most likely explanation has to do with hormones. We make oestrogens in our body fat, so the more fat we have, the more oestrogen exposure we get and the higher our breast cancer risk. Exercise probably protects against colon cancer by helping to speed wastes through the digestive tract. This gives carcinogens less time to act on the lining of the colon.

Arthritis and Joint Problems

About 6–8 million Britons suffer from some form of arthritis, diseases of the joints. Excess weight is often a contributing factor, especially in osteoarthritis: the joints of the ankles, knees and hips don't get any larger if you gain weight, but they have to work a lot harder. People who suffer from arthritis often lose muscle and become weaker, not only because their mobility is impaired but also because of the medications they take. In the past, people with arthritis were advised not to exercise, for fear of causing pain and further damage to the joints. However, several important new studies have shown that both strength training and aerobic exercise not only are safe but also provide pain relief, and improve mobility and strength.

Osteoporosis

This devastating condition, in which bones become dangerously fragile, mostly affects women over the age of 50. But preventive measures should be taken by women several decades younger. The more bone mass a woman can accumulate before menopause, the larger her reserves later in life.

For someone with osteoporosis, an accidental fall can mean broken bones, disability, and even death. Indeed, more women die each year from hip fractures related to osteoporosis than from breast cancer, uterine cancer, and ovarian cancer combined! My JAMA study showed that strength training just two times a week dramatically cuts the risk of osteoporosis by restoring bone, building strength, and improving balance, thereby reducing the risk of falls. Other research has demonstrated that weight-bearing aerobic activities, such as calisthenics and walking, are also beneficial. We don't yet have long-term data on osteoporosis risk in women who do both strength training *and* aerobic exercise. But my guess is that they will enjoy the greatest protection of all.

ACTIVE WOMEN ARE HAPPIER

I'm a secretary, and I sit in front of a computer all day. I've finally started to understand my body when it tells me I need to exercise. I might be a little depressed and I know that if I take a walk, I'll feel better. Or I get stiff and crabby at the same time, and I make the connection—my body is telling me to do something.
        —Therese

♦ ♦ ♦

My favourite way to unwind after a hectic week is to go into the woods behind our house and take a long walk. No matter how much tension has built up, after a brisk walk I feel peaceful and relaxed. Research suggests that many women have the same response to exercise. There's evidence that physical activity enhances mood, improves coping skills, and boosts self-esteem and self-confidence. Active people are only half as likely as their sedentary counterparts to suffer from the bouts of anxiety and depression that are so prevalent in our modern world.

All this is especially good news for a woman who finds herself turning to food in response to stress or unhappiness—and then feeling worse because she gains weight. Exercise gives her a way to get unstuck.

BEING ACTIVE MAKES WOMEN FEEL BETTER ABOUT THEMSELVES

Self-esteem and self-confidence are the fundamentals of mental health. Do you like yourself? Do you believe you can accomplish what you want to do? For many overweight women, the answer is "No". For starters, problems with self-esteem and self-confidence are more common in women than in men. Excess weight adds to the emotional burden. Looking back on how she felt before she started strength training, Martha told me:

> *I avoided going to social events because I wasn't pleased with what I looked like and my clothes didn't fit. I didn't feel good about myself. I wasn't proud of myself. I had a problem I wasn't dealing with, so I felt out of control.*

Exercise turns these feelings around almost immediately. When women lose weight as well, the transformation is almost magical. Martha says:

> *I take such pleasure in my progress—more pleasure and more comfort than I used to find in food. I feel in control and I'm happier about everything.*

Fitness Fights Depression

Some people get such a delightful boost from vigorous exercise that they describe themselves as feeling high. Actually, they may not be wrong. As mentioned in Chapter 2, scientists speculate that aerobic exercise improves mood by stimulating production of endorphins, chemicals in the brain that have effects similar to those of opiates. Indeed, the word "endorphin" comes from the same root as "morphine".

We've known for years about the depression-fighting benefits of aerobic exercise. Now we're learning that strength training is equally helpful. A study done in our laboratory by Nalin Singh, MD, and colleagues looked at 32 men and women who suffered from chronic depression. Half the volunteers did strength training; the others simply received health education. Twelve weeks later, 14 out of the 16 members of the strength training group felt so much better that they no longer met the clinical criteria for depression, but only 6 members of the education-only group enjoyed similar relief. This impressive success rate is comparable to that produced by highly effective anti-depressants.

Physical Activity Reduces Anxiety and Stress

Many women tell me—and research confirms—that one of the best benefits of exercise is that their stress levels have dropped. They feel calmer and more relaxed in general. Also, they now turn to exercise rather than to food when they face stress-provoking situations.

◆   ◆   ◆

I go to a massage therapist because of tension in my neck and right shoulder. After I started strength training, she noticed that my whole upper body seemed more opened up. My shoulders were held back naturally, and I didn't have that round-shouldered look.
—Jane

◆   ◆   ◆

Exercise Is Better Than a Sleeping Pill

Active people have more energy during the day, and they sleep better at night. In scientific studies, many measures of sleep quality show improvements: people who get regular exercise fall asleep more quickly, sleep more deeply, awaken less often in the middle of the night, and sleep longer. These benefits are comparable to those of medication, but with none of the side effects.

Now that researchers are exploring the effects of strength training, we're finding similar results. In Dr Singh's study of depression, 10 people in the strength-training group and 7 in the health-education group reported sleep problems when they joined the project. After 12 weeks, 6 of the 10 strength-training volunteers reported that they no longer had difficulty sleeping; in contrast, no one in the health-education group improved.

A LITTLE BIT MAKES A BIG DIFFERENCE

You might assume that adding a little exercise would give you just a little benefit. That's true for those who are already exercising vigorously—

doing more doesn't make a big difference for health. But small changes can have major effects for sedentary people. In Dr Blair's research at the Cooper Institute for Aerobics Research, which I described earlier in this chapter, the most dramatic drop in mortality came when people changed from being totally sedentary to being moderately active. **The more inactive you are now, the more you will benefit from exercise.**

Strength training delivers significant improvements with just two or three 30-minute sessions per week. For aerobic exercise, three to five 30-minute workouts per week suffice. You don't even have to engage in planned exercise to benefit. Dr Blair and others have shown that simply being more active in everyday life—walking more, climbing more stairs, spending more time on active hobbies like gardening and golf—improves health and reduces mortality.

The *Strong Women Stay Slim* programme will gently ease you into a more active lifestyle. Strength training and aerobic exercise will help you lose weight and keep it off. But the beauty of exercise is that it does so much more. Because you're reducing the risk of many chronic diseases and disabilities, you're increasing the odds that you'll live a long and healthy life. The benefits begin immediately, even before you shed a kilogram. You'll have a surge of energy and a tremendous sense of pride in what you're accomplishing. So you'll feel healthier and happier right from the start.

EATING FOR HEALTH

AND PLEASURE

I need a lot of flexibility. This plan allowed me to eat well, to make choices, and to give myself a treat. If I really wanted butter on my bread, I could have it. If I baked cookies with the kids, I could eat one. I could have a drink before dinner. It made all the difference to me that I had the leeway and the freedom.

— Nancy

◆ ◆ ◆

On Sunday mornings I serve waffles for breakfast, a wonderful tradition from my husband's family. Guests who join us for the first time often are surprised to see me—a dietitian—piling my plate with waffles and fruit, and topping the stack with sour cream and maple syrup. But there's nothing wrong with this meal. It's a perfectly reasonable part of the well-rounded diet and active lifestyle that keep me and my family healthy and slender. Even with this indulgence, our weekly consumption of fats and sweets is within guidelines for good nutrition. During the rest of the day we more than compensate for the extra calories with vigorous physical activity.

The best way to lose weight is through a combination of exercise and a wholesome food plan that lets you take pleasure in eating again. Good nutrition becomes particularly important when you're trying to lose weight. Not only do you need to select the right foods for weight loss, you also want to be sure they deliver the essentials you need. Scientists now know a great deal about the optimal diet for health and longevity. But only you can determine how to adapt this information to your life and your preferences—and that's a key part of staying slim. Yes, you can lose weight on a diet you don't like. But how will you maintain the loss? A food plan you enjoy is one you will follow for a lifetime.

EATING SHOULD BE A PLEASURE

When I sit down for a meal with women friends and relatives, I'm often dismayed to hear comments like these:

> *I shouldn't be eating this.*
> *I've wrecked the whole week with this meal.*

For many women, eating is fraught with guilt and unhappiness. Instead of savouring the delicious food served on special occasions—family gatherings, dinner parties with friends, and holiday celebrations at the office—they worry about losing control and eating too much. A tiny bit of guilt is a superb motivator, but beyond that it's counterproductive. When you feel guilty about food, it's easy to fall into a negative spiral of self-criticism, poor self-image, and even depression—which leads to overeating and more bad feelings. This is one reason that overly restrictive diets seldom work in the long run.

When you need to control the *quantity* of food you eat, it becomes even more important to enjoy the *quality*. The pleasure that you get from eating is a significant part of life. You don't have to turn your back on it; rather, you have to harness this potent motivator. Here are three basic principles for maximising enjoyment as you lose weight:

♦ EAT TO THE LIMIT

You can't lose weight unless your calorie intake is consistently less than your calorie expenditure. But the gap should be as small as possible while still allowing you to lose. It's not just a matter of minimising deprivation, though that's a very important goal. The more you eat, the more nutrients your diet can provide, and the healthier and more satisfying it will be. As you may have experienced yourself, women who cut back too much can send their body into starvation mode, thwarting their efforts to lose. Their metabolic rate drops, they become lethargic and therefore burn fewer calories through physical activity, and their appetite screams for food.

♦ INCLUDE YOUR FAVOURITE FOODS

I'm not saying you're going to be able to eat any amount of everything you might want. But if you take great pleasure in certain foods, it's important to have them in appropriate quantities so you don't feel deprived.

One woman on our programme, Lillian, sometimes says that the secret of her successful weight loss is peanut butter. She'd been slim all her life, then went through a difficult period in her early fifties and gained 9 kilograms (20 lb). When she finally decided to go on a diet, she wanted quick results. She selected a plan that had worked well for a friend, even though it prohibited peanut butter and other foods she enjoys. She lost the 9 kilograms (20 lb) in just three months—but a year later the weight was back. After several more yo-yo cycles she came to me. "I rebound on peanut butter," she said. "I love it, but I know I shouldn't eat it because it's so fattening."

"If you enjoy peanut butter, there's no reason you can't have it," I told her. We worked out nutritious meal plans that included reasonable portions of peanut butter and her other favourites. Six months later, Lillian's excess weight was gone—and she's maintained the loss for three years.

♦ CULTIVATE NEW PREFERENCES

When you're losing weight, it's not enough to restrict calories—it's also important to eat a healthy variety of foods so you get all the nutrients your body needs. An astonishing abundance is available in stores and produce markets today, but we sometimes limit ourselves to what's familiar. Alexandra,

WHERE DO FOOD CRAVINGS COME FROM?

Cravings sometimes reflect actual physical needs, either for specific nutrients or for food in general. Though we don't yet have solid research on this, many clinical dietitians have noticed that when their clients begin eating a varied, well-balanced diet and get enough food, their cravings are greatly reduced.

Another source of cravings is emotional. We associate certain foods with comfort or good times, so we may yearn for them when we're under stress. Adding to this effect is the fact that high-carbohydrate foods increase the brain's supply of serotonin, a naturally occurring mood-elevating chemical.

told me that sweets were her downfall. A few weeks after she started the programme, when we discussed her food diary, I congratulated her on cutting back her dessert portions. But I also noted that her fruit consumption was limited to orange juice, raisins, and apples. "I've never liked fruit," she explained. "Besides, it's too much trouble to prepare." I suggested she try one new fruit per week. She agreed to start with ready-to-eat melon chunks from the salad bar at her supermarket.

One year and 21 kilograms (46 lb) later, Alexandra's tastes had expanded considerably. She recently e-mailed me this update:

> We had friends over the other night, and I served fresh pineapple and gateau. The pineapple was so luscious that I took seconds and ignored the gateau. Afterward, when I realised what I'd done, I was absolutely stunned: I've become one of those people who eats fruit for dessert!

CALORIES ALWAYS COUNT

One way or another, *all* weight reduction diets restrict food energy so that intake is lower than energy expenditure. Some keep track of calories. Others—including the food plan in this book—focus on portions instead, but that's just a simpler way to count calories.

A less obvious way to restrict calories is to limit your food choices. Some "calories don't count" plans limit dieters to just a few specific foods; others rule out entire categories. The secret of their temporary success is that most people get bored with the permitted foods, and they eat less. However, that very same boredom makes the diet all but impossible to follow for a lifetime, so the weight returns.

GOOD NUTRITION FOR WEIGHT LOSS

Any diet that cuts enough calories can produce weight loss. I hope you're looking for a lot more—good nutrition, practicality, flexibility, and enjoyment. These are the considerations I keep in mind when I review research about the best diets for weight control.

The food plan in this book, which I'll detail in Chapter 9, is based on the United States Food Guide Pyramid. This blueprint for nutritious eating distills decades of research about the relationship between diet and longevity and optimum health—large-scale surveys, as well as meticulous laboratory investigations. British equivalents (produced by the Health Education Authority) are very similar.

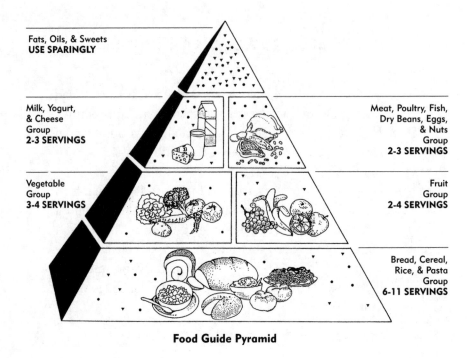

Fats, Oils, & Sweets
USE SPARINGLY

Milk, Yogurt,
& Cheese
Group
2-3 SERVINGS

Meat, Poultry, Fish,
Dry Beans, Eggs,
& Nuts
Group
2-3 SERVINGS

Vegetable
Group
3-4 SERVINGS

Fruit
Group
2-4 SERVINGS

Bread, Cereal,
Rice, & Pasta
Group
6-11 SERVINGS

Food Guide Pyramid

In Chapter 9 I'll show you how to translate these guidelines into daily menus that give you all the nutrients you need. And there's plenty of room for adjustments to allow for your preferences.

THE ESSENTIAL INGREDIENTS

The *Strong Women Stay Slim* food plan optimises the Food Guide Pyramid for weight loss, while retaining as much flexibility as possible. While you're losing weight you'll be well nourished. Afterwards, you can use the same structure for a lifetime of healthy eating. Let's look individually at the basic components that this plan provides.

CARBOHYDRATES

Many women are confused about carbohydrates—and no wonder. Some experts recommend that you eat them in abundance when you're dieting, while others warn that you must carefully limit them to lose weight. Women often ask me questions about high-carbohydrate foods:

Will pasta make me fat?
Should I be eating potatoes?
Is it bad to have bread?

Most dietitians—including me—consider carbohydrates the staff of life. They're the body's chief source of fuel, providing most of the energy we need for exercise and everything else we do. Carbohydrates also play an important role in satisfying our appetite: as they're converted into sugar and enter the blood stream, they signal to the hypothalamus that we've eaten.

THE GLYCAEMIC INDEX

The glycaemic index is a measure of how rapidly the carbohydrates in a food are broken down and turned into sugar in the blood. You may have heard about weight-loss approaches that feature a blanket recommendation against foods that have a high glycaemic index. There's no scientific basis for avoiding all such foods—a list that would include carrots, bananas, potatoes, pasta, and wholegrain bread. On the contrary, there's plenty of evidence to suggest that these items are good for you. They supply valuable nutrients, and scientific surveys show that people who consume a diet high in these complex carbohydrates enjoy above-average health. However, certain high-glycaemic foods, like chocolate, provide nothing but calories. It's also true that a diet with a large amount of high-glycaemic foods *plus* a low fibre intake can put you at risk for heart disease and diabetes. And, of course, any food can cause weight gain if consumed in excess.

When you follow the food plan in this book, about 55 to 60 per cent of the calories you consume will be from carbohydrates.

There are two kinds of carbohydrates in food: sugars and starches. On their own, sugars add only flavour and calories to our diet—that's why the Food Guide Pyramid recommends that they be eaten sparingly. This is just as true for "natural" or "unrefined" forms like honey or maple syrup as it is for cane sugar. But you can more freely indulge your sweet tooth with the sugars in fruit because they come with valuable extras. For instance, the sugar in an orange is accompanied by impressive amounts of fibre, vitamin C, folate, potassium and other valuable nutrients.

Starches—better known these days as "complex carbohydrates"—are found in grains, legumes (peas, beans), potatoes, and other vegetables. Your body has to work harder to digest starch than sugar; this is especially true when the starch is in unrefined grains, because those also contain fibre. That's an advantage when you're trying to lose weight: the slower a food is metabolised, the longer your appetite will feel satisfied. Furthermore, whole grains provide important trace minerals that aren't found in many other foods.

PROTEIN

Protein is the body's chief building material—our muscles, bones, cartilage, skin, hair and blood are made in part from protein. When you follow the food plan in this book, 15 to 20 per cent of your calorie intake is from protein.

We use many different kinds of protein, but all are combinations of the same twenty amino acids. Our body manufactures eleven of these acids, but the other nine—the essential amino acids—must be obtained from food. It's easy to get enough if you eat animal products: meat, poultry, seafood, eggs, and dairy foods are rich in protein. Of course, low-fat versions are best for weight loss.

Certain plant foods contain protein too, but these proteins lack one or more of the nine essential amino acids. Fortunately for vegetarians, different plants contain different amino acids. Well-chosen combinations—including traditional favourites such as rice and beans or corn and beans—can provide a complete set.

The question I'm most frequently asked about protein is this:

If protein helps build muscle, can extra protein give me added muscle and strength?

There's no scientific evidence that it can. One of my colleagues, Wayne Campbell, Ph.D., investigated this question in a careful study that was published in the *American Journal of Clinical Nutrition* in 1994. Twelve men and women volunteered to spend twelve weeks living in our metabolic unit at Tufts, so that everything they ate and everything they excreted could be measured. Half of them consumed the recommended amount of protein, and half were given a diet with double that amount. The volunteers also did vigorous strength training to build muscles. The extra dietary protein had no effect. At the end of twelve weeks, there was no difference between the two groups in muscle tissue and strength. Other studies have since corroborated this finding.

THE PROBLEM WITH HIGH-PROTEIN/ LOW-CARBOHYDRATE DIETS

If you cut carbohydrates drastically and add a corresponding amount of protein, your body is forced to turn to an inferior fuel source: protein metabolites called ketones. Because ketones are toxic, your kidneys go into overdrive to flush them out of your system. In the process, you drain water from your tissues. Since a litre (2 pints) of water weighs about a kilogram (2 lb), you can lose a lot of weight very quickly on a high-protein/low-carbohydrate diet. And you may drop an additional kilogram or two because you're eating less.

There's good news on the scales, perhaps, but bad news for your body. You've lost mainly water—along with calcium from your bones and protein from your muscles—but not as much fat as you think. Moreover, your kidneys are under stress; you may become dehydrated, which puts an extra strain on your heart. Many women become weak after a week or more on a ketogenic diet. Their heart may race or they may become dizzy from minor exertion; they often develop bad breath and other problems. Few people can—or should—stay on this kind of diet in the long run. The weight usually returns quickly as the body's water supply is restored.

Fat

If you're trying to lose weight you may think of fat as the enemy, but that's not quite fair. We all need fat in our diet. Fat supplies two essential nutrients—linoleic acid and linolenic acid —that are necessary for the formation of prostaglandins, which are hormone-like compounds that help control reproduction, blood pressure, and other important functions. Fat is also important for appetite control. Because it's broken down more slowly than carbohydrate and protein, it keeps you feeling full longer after a meal. Fat also carries flavour and improves texture, making many foods more enjoyable. On this food plan, about 25 per cent of your daily calorie intake is from fat.

Getting enough dietary fat is easy because so many foods contain fat. There's fat in oils and butter, obviously, and in most sources of protein and in dairy foods; grains and legumes also contain small amounts.

Fat becomes a problem when we eat too much of it. Unfortunately, that's easy to do. Fat is more calorie-dense than protein or carbohydrate—nine calories per gram compared with four. That's why a scoop of high-fat ice cream might have twice as many calories as the same size portion of low-fat

NON-FAT DOESN'T MEAN NON-FATTENING!

Food manufacturers have done a terrific job of cutting back on excess fat in processed foods. For instance, low-fat and non-fat dairy products allow us to get all the nutritional benefits of milk, yoghurt, and cheese, without excessive fat. But you can't assume that all no-fat foods are healthy, or that they're low in calories.

Like many dietitians, I've been concerned by the proliferation of snacks and desserts that are "non-fat," but high-sugar and high-calorie. Some women consume these products freely, then wonder why they don't lose weight. But very often the non-fat version has just about the same number of calories as the regular version—and sometimes even more.

yoghurt. Excess food does more damage when it's high in fat. That's because your body can convert *dietary* fat into *stored* fat with very little metabolic effort. Turning 100 extra carbohydrate calories into body fat "costs" 23 calories, so only 77 calories actually get stored. But if the excess 100 calories come from fat, the process is far more efficient and requires only 3 calories—which means that 97 calories become body fat.

Dietary fat can be a problem even for people who are not overweight, because it affects blood chemistry and can lead to heart disease and stroke. Certain kinds of fat are more harmful than others, so it's good to be selective.

- ◆ **Saturated fats**—the kind that are solid at room temperature, like butter, lard, and palm oil—come from animal and dairy products, plus a few plants. People whose diet is high in saturated fat tend to have higher levels of both LDL and HDL cholesterol. (See box on cholesterol.)

What About Cholesterol?

Cholesterol is essential to life—but it's become almost synonymous with heart disease because it can clog the arteries, leading to heart attack and stroke. The liver manufactures cholesterol, and most of us get extra cholesterol from food. All fat of animal origin—including egg yolks, dairy fat, and the fat from meat and poultry—contains cholesterol; there's none in fat that comes from plants, such as cocoa butter, or olive or peanut oil.

In the bloodstream, cholesterol is piggy-backed on proteins called **lipoproteins. Low-density lipoproteins (LDL)** bring cholesterol to the cells, but they also deposit it on the arteries. For that reason, LDL is called "bad cholesterol". In contrast, the job of the **high-density lipoproteins (HDL)**—"good cholesterol"—is to remove cholesterol from the bloodstream. (To remember the difference, think H for healthy and L for ill.)

- **Trans fatty acid** is vegetable oil that's been made solid by a manufacturing process called hydrogenation. (Look for "hydrogenated vegetable oil" on the label.) It's very similar to saturated fat. That's why, nutritionally speaking, there's not much difference between butter and solid margarine.

- **Monounsaturated fat** is liquid at room temperature, but becomes partly firm if chilled. Many experts believe that you can lower LDL and increase HDL by substituting monounsaturated fat for saturated fat—for example, dipping your bread in olive oil instead of spreading it with butter.

- **Polyunsaturated fat** remains liquid unless you put it in the freezer. The fat in most vegetable oils is polyunsaturated, as is the fat in cold-water fish, whose fat must stay liquid so the fish can move. These fats seem to be heart-friendly. An added benefit of vegetable oils is that they contain vitamin E, which I'll discuss later in this chapter.

Dietary Fibre

Fibre is one of nature's best appetite suppressants: it fills you up—yet it contains no calories. Plus, fibre sweeps waste through your gastrointestinal tract. This not only prevents constipation and related ills, but also lowers your risk of colon cancer because carcinogens have less time to act on the intestinal lining. Fibre even provides benefits to the heart, since it helps remove cholesterol from the small intestines. The food plan in this book, which calls for plenty of fruits and vegetables, provides ample fibre.

There are two types of fibre, both of which are valuable for health and satiety:

- **Soluble fibre**, which can absorb water, turning into a soft gel; it's found in fruits, legumes, oats, rye, and barley.

- **Insoluble fibre**, which doesn't absorb water; sources include whole-wheat products, bran, and fruit and vegetable skins.

Most people in the western world don't get enough fibre—but that doesn't mean you should sprinkle bran on your food. In excessive quantities, fibre speeds helpful substances—including essential minerals such as calcium, iron, and zinc—out of the body before they can be absorbed. Also, too much fibre can irritate the bowel. However, when fibre is consumed as part of whole foods, it's almost impossible to get too much.

WATER

Water is another important weight-loss aid. Though it contains no calories, it contributes to fullness. Many women have told me that they're satisfied with smaller portions when they sip water along with a meal. But that's just one reason it's important to drink enough when you're trying to take off weight. The body uses water for most of its behind-the-scenes processes, from digesting food to sweating. You probably know that you need extra water when you exercise. It's also very important for maintaining energy throughout the day. Many people who feel lethargic don't realise that the reason isn't always lack of sleep; rather, they may be slightly dehydrated. That's why a glass of cool water can be a surprisingly helpful pick-me-up. The *Strong Women Stay Slim* food plan recommends that you drink at least eight glasses of water or other fluids per day.

ALCOHOL

If alcohol were on the Food Guide Pyramid, it would be in the "use sparingly" category because of the calories it contains. In moderate quantities, alcoholic beverages (especially red wine) appear to increase HDL, which makes them heart-friendly. However, excessive alcohol consumption causes many problems, including nutritional deficiencies—not only because alcohol substitutes for more nutritious food, but also because it damages the liver and interferes with the metabolism of many nutrients.

MINERALS AND VITAMINS

When you follow the food plan in this book, you get all the vitamins and minerals you need. These nutrients contain no calories, but they're essential to good health.

Our teeth and bones are made up of minerals—mainly calcium, but also phosphorus, magnesium, and fluoride. Minerals also are involved in many of the chemical reactions that sustain life, including metabolism, muscle contractions, and the transmission of nerve impulses.

Vitamins contribute to the body's biochemical functioning as well. Thanks to improved diet, including vitamin-enriched grains, we rarely encounter the deficiencies that were once a common cause of disability and death. However, as I'll discuss later in this chapter, we're beginning to learn that some vitamins have additional health-promoting potential if consumed in larger amounts than we typically get from food.

SURPRISING BONUSES FROM FOOD

The Food Guide Pyramid recommends a diet with plenty of fruits, vegetables, and whole grains. That's because large comparative studies have found that people who follow such a diet are healthier and live longer. We don't know all the reasons, but it's clear that vitamins and minerals are only part of the explanation. I'm tremendously excited by a discovery that is still unfolding: that plant foods contain *thousands* of health-promoting chemicals called **phytochemicals** (from the Greek word "phyto" meaning "plant"). Consider them yet another benefit you'll get from the food plan in this book.

One type of phytochemical of particular interest to women are **isoflavones**, also known as phyto-oestrogens—plant oestrogens. Isoflavones, which are found in soybeans, are similar to the oestrogens produced by your body. They may explain why Asian women, who consume far more soy than British women do, have fewer hip fractures and fewer menopausal symptoms—in fact, there's no equivalent of "hot flushes" in some Asian languages. Many British women take hormone replacement therapy (HRT) to counter problems associated with menopause; unfortunately, the advantages of HRT

ANTIOXIDANTS

People don't rust, and we don't spoil the way food can, but our cells are similarly damaged by the same chemical process: **oxidation**. This damage is now believed to be partly responsible for cancer and many degenerative conditions associated with ageing, from cataracts to wrinkles. I'll explain how it happens.

During normal chemical reactions in the body, cells produce oxygen compounds. Some of these compounds are unstable because they're missing an electron. These unbalanced molecules—called free radicals—take electrons from other molecules, which then become unbalanced themselves. This chain reaction of molecular change is what breaks down healthy material during oxidation. Free radicals are produced by normal processes, and also by air pollution, cigarette smoke, and other stresses to the body.

Harmful oxidation is kept in check by substances called **antioxidants**. These have the ability to donate an electron without becoming unduly unstable, so they can neutralise a free radical without creating more. The body produces its own antioxidants, but we also need some from the foods we eat. Antioxidant nutrients include vitamin C, vitamin E, and numerous phytochemicals.

are counterbalanced by a small increase in the risk of breast cancer. But Asian women get similar benefits from soy, *and* they have very low breast cancer rates. How come? Apparently the isoflavones in soybeans are a less potent form of oestrogen, so they're less likely to stimulate tumours in breast tissue.

In the table on the next two pages, I summarise just a few of the promising phytochemicals and the magic they appear to work. As you'll see, a wide variety of fruits, vegetables, legumes, herbs, and grains contribute. How can you possibly take advantage of this natural pharmacy when we don't even know its full extent? The best way is to consume a rainbow of plant-based foods.

PHYTO-CHEMICAL	WHAT IT APPEARS TO DO	BEST FOOD SOURCES
Isoflavones (also known as phyto-oestrogens)	Reduce risk of breast and ovarian cancer, and osteoporosis; also relieve hot flushes and other symptoms of menopuase	Soybeans and dried beans
Flavonoids	Reduce risk of heart disease by decreasing oxidation of LDL cholesterol	Red wine, apples, celery, cranberries, grapes, black and green tea, onions
Lutein and zeaxanthin (found together in foods)	Reduce risk of macular degeneration, the leading cause of blindness in older people	Yellow, orange, and dark green leafy vegetables
Ellagic acid	Reduce activity of carcinogens found in tobacco and environmental pollutants	Grapes, strawberries, raspberries
Allyl sulphides	Reduce cancer risk by helping to neutralise carcinogens; also may interfere with reproduction of tumour cells	Garlic, onions, leeks, chives

Phyto-chemical	What It Appears to Do	Best Food Sources
Terpenes	Block development of cancer tumours (tamoxifen and taxol, which are used to treat breast cancer, are both terpenes)	Citrus fruits
Isothiocyanates	Trigger the formation of enzymes that could prevent carcinogens from damaging DNA	Cruciferous vegetables like broccoli, cabbage, and cauliflower
Indoles	Reduce the risk of breast cancer by helping the body convert a potentially harmful form of oestrogen into a harmless form	Cruciferous vegetables like broccoli, cabbage, and cauliflower
Saponins	Prevent cancer cells from multiplying	Soybeans and other dried beans, cherries
Lycopene	Decreases risk of prostate cancer, probably by reducing DNA damage from oxidation of cells. May decrease other cancers for women	Tomatoes (for lycopene to be absorbed, it must be consumed with some fat)

DO WE NEED SUPPLEMENTS?

As a dietitian, I'm asked about supplements all the time, not only in the office and at lectures, but also by family and friends. The question isn't easy to answer, because it takes years of research to prove that a supplement provides real benefits and has no harmful side effects. Until recently I never thought about taking supplements myself or recommending them to others, except during pregnancy. Instead I'd suggest consuming a wide variety of wholesome foods. After all, pills can't possibly replace a well-rounded diet because there are so many unknown beneficial components of food— especially all those phytochemicals. However, I'm beginning to reconsider. New research suggests that even people who choose their foods carefully might benefit from additional amounts of certain nutrients.

CALCIUM

We all know that our bones are made from calcium, and that a high-calcium diet helps keep them strong. But not everyone realises that calcium is also an essential part of the body's biochemistry: it's needed for contraction of muscles (including the heart), for blood clotting and for nerve conduction. Indeed, calcium is so important that if we don't get enough in our diet, our body is forced to draw it from our bones.

Just how much is enough for optimal bone health? This is the subject of some controversy, but current evidence supports the new dietary calcium RDAs: 800 milligrams (mg) daily for women aged 19 to 54; 1000 mg for women over 54; and 1300 mg for women who are breastfeeding. If you decide to take a calcium supplement, choose a dose that reflects what you're already consuming in your diet. If you follow the food plan in this book, which includes two or three servings of dairy foods, your daily calcium intake will be around 700 to 800 milligrams per day; a sufficient supplement would be 300 mg if you're 50 or under, or 500 mg if you're older, or 600 mg if you're breast-feeding.

VITAMIN D

Calcium gets all the attention, but vitamin D is equally important: without this vitamin your body can't effectively use the calcium you consume. We get vitamin D from food and from the sun, which stimulates our skin cells to manufacture it. All you need is 10 minutes of full sunlight to get your daily supply, but that may not be possible in the winter, so I suggest a supplement that supplies 400 to 700 international units (IU) (but don't go above 1000 IU, because vitamin D is toxic at high levels).

A BONE-FRIENDLY COMBINATION: CALCIUM PLUS VITAMIN D

We've known for a long time that taking calcium supplements plus vitamin D can slow bone loss after menopause. Now two important studies—one by French investigators and another by my colleague Bess Dawson-Hughes, M.D., and associates at Tufts—have shown that this combination translates into impressive reductions in hip and other bone fractures. Dr Dawson-Hughes's investigation followed 389 elderly men and women for three years. About half of the volunteers were given a daily supplement containing 500 milligrams of calcium and 700 international units of vitamin D; the rest received a placebo. During the three years, men and women in the two groups were about equally likely to fall. But only 6 per cent of those taking the supplements suffered a fracture, compared with 13 per cent of those who were merely getting a placebo. This remarkable benefit is comparable to the effects of hormone replacement therapy and other medications used to treat osteoporosis.

FOLATE

If you've been pregnant any time in the past twenty years, you may have been told to take a vitamin supplement high in folate (also called folic acid), one of the B vitamins. Folate plays a key role in the development of the nervous system; a deficiency during pregnancy increases the risk of nervous system birth defects. More recently we've learned that folate may help prevent heart disease, stroke, and declining mental functioning in the elderly, since it helps control a substance in the blood called homocysteine. (See box.) Also, there's some evidence that low folate intake could be a factor in colon cancer.

It's possible to get adequate folate from the diet, but many women don't consume enough folate-rich foods. Sources include liver, dark green leafy vegetables, broccoli, oranges, beans, and peas. If your diet is low in folate and you decide to take a supplement, 400 micrograms per day is adequate. Select a supplement that also includes 2 milligrams of vitamin B-6 and 2 to 5 micrograms of vitamin B-12, since all three of these nutrients work together.

CORONARY DISEASE: THE HOMOCYSTEINE CONNECTION

When the body processes methionine, an amino acid, one of the byproducts is homocysteine. In order to break it down we need folate, a B vitamin. If we don't get enough, homocysteine may accumulate in the blood. Excessive homocysteine can damage the lining of the arteries, making them more vulnerable to cholesterol deposits.

Attention was drawn to homocysteine more than twenty-five years ago, when a Harvard physician autopsied an 8-year-old boy who had died of a stroke. The child had plaque-choked arteries—and abnormally high homocysteine levels. More recent studies at Tufts by Jacob Selhub, Ph.D., and colleagues found that individuals with elevated amounts of homocysteine in their blood had *triple* the average risk of heart attack. Others have corroborated these findings. Genetic factors appear to affect homocysteine levels. But Dr Selhub estimates that at least two-thirds of elevated homocysteine can be explained by inadequate intake of folate and of vitamins B-6 and B-12.

VITAMIN C

Vitamin C is a potent antioxidant—indeed, it's sometimes added to food as a preservative—so we've hoped it might act against disease. Dozens of studies have tried to prove that vitamin C can prevent the common cold, but all we know for sure is that it may help shorten the duration and severity of a cold once you've caught it. However, there's persuasive research evidence that vitamin C can help protect against two common causes of vision problems in the elderly: cataracts and macular degeneration. Seven different studies have shown that a daily intake of at least 300 mg of vitamin C is associated with a reduction of up to 70 per cent in cataracts. It's possible to get 300 mg if you eat plenty of fruits and vegetables, which also give you many other nutrients. If you plan to take a vitamin C supplement, I recommend taking between 200 and 300 mg per day.

VITAMIN E

This vitamin—found in wheat germ, vegetable oils, and nuts—is a potent antioxidant. Half of Britons don't meet the current RDA for vitamin E, and evidence is accumulating that supplements above the RDA may provide additional health benefits.

My Tufts colleague Simin Meydani, D.V.M., Ph.D., recently published promising findings about vitamin E in the *Journal of the American Medical Association*. She and her associates demonstrated that elderly men and women who took vitamin E supplements for four months showed a 50 per cent improvement in several indexes of immune function. Others have found an association between vitamin E supplements and decreased colon cancer, stroke, and Alzheimer's disease. One intriguing English study found that men and women who already suffered from heart disease had 70 per cent fewer heart attacks when they took vitamin E. The investigators speculate that oxidised LDLs are the ones most likely to deposit cholesterol in arteries, and that vitamin E prevents them from becoming oxidised. Can vitamin E help younger people too? Possibly, though the benefits seem to be less dramatic. The recommended amount for vitamin E supplementation is 100 to 400 international units daily.

If you're like most weight-conscious women, you've probably made many health-promoting changes in your diet already. The food plan in this book will help you make more, not just for the months during which you're losing weight but for the rest of your life. Eating well will make you happier, healthier, and more energetic—and you'll look better too.

II

GETTING
STARTED

5

THE SEVEN MENTAL SECRETS OF SUCCESSFUL WEIGHT LOSS

I used to go on a diet every Monday, and also on the first of each month, on January 2 (after our annual New Year's open house), and on the day after my birthday—unless there was cake left over, in which case I'd put it off. There was dieting and there was real life. Until now I had no idea how to make them work together.
—Alexandra

◆ ◆ ◆

When I was in my twenties I was a competitive marathoner. When I meet a woman who's starting a weight-loss programme, I'm struck by how similar her task is to running a marathon. Both require long, hard work despite the fact that the finish line is far away. Success depends on the ability to sustain motivation and focus. That's why weight loss isn't just a matter of diet and exercise. A lot of brainwork is required too.

The mental secrets of successful weight loss aren't really different from the mental secrets of being an athlete, quitting smoking, or taking on any other difficult personal challenge. That's why, when I work with women who want to lose weight, I draw upon seemingly unrelated fields, such as sports psychology and smoking cessation. You probably have most of the necessary mental skills already—if not, you can easily learn them. As you do, you'll find they apply to many areas of your life. When you succeed in losing weight, you will realise that you can succeed in anything.

SECRET #1: BELIEVE THAT YOU CAN DO IT

I'm always concerned when I hear a woman put herself down with statements like these:

I'm lazy—I'll never be able to exercise.
I don't have the self-control to follow a food plan.

I believe that we actually listen when we talk to ourselves. Just as we benefit from the supportive words of a loving friend or relative, we need to hear our own encouraging messages. Judith told me:

I find affirmations very helpful. These are strong, positive statements that I make to myself several times a day. One is: "I am a slender, healthy, energetic, strong, and vibrant woman living my life with grace, ease, and balance." I don't say I wish I could be like this. I say the affirmation as if the changes had already happened.

Believing in yourself really makes a difference. There is dramatic evidence from a 1996 University of Maryland study involving 54 women who followed a diet and exercise programme for nine months. Before they started, investigators asked them whether they thought they'd lose weight. Twenty-eight of the women were "believers" and 26 were "disbelievers." The believers expected to get trim—and they did. At the end of nine months they'd lost 30 per cent more weight than those who lacked faith in themselves.

You may feel sceptical. Perhaps you've tried dieting before without results; or you've lost weight only to regain it. Then there's the widely quoted "fact" that more than 90 per cent of those who try to lose weight permanently

BECOMING A BELIEVER:
THE POWER OF VISUALISATION

These days no serious athlete trains without the help of visualisation. You can use the same technique to help with weight loss. It's easy to learn, simple to do—and remarkably powerful.

Though you can do visualisation anywhere, it helps to find a place where you can sit comfortably without being interrupted. Relax, close your eyes, and picture yourself succeeding. Let your mind conjure up as many details as possible. See yourself accomplishing the task step by step.

◆ **Motivate** yourself by visualising the changes you're working to achieve.

I try on my favourite blue suit, which I haven't worn since my pregnancy—and it fits! Wearing the suit, I walk into a meeting at work, aware that I'm standing tall and looking attractive.

◆ **Prepare** for the day ahead by visualising what you're going to do.

I change into walking shoes, and I drink a glass of water. At the park, I move slowly at first, then gradually speed up. I walk briskly along the path, swinging my arms. Afterward, my body feels energised and warm.

◆ **Troubleshoot** by visualising yourself managing a difficult situation.

My sister-in-law serves me a slice of chocolate layer cake. I take one bite, and tell her how delicious it is. Then I put my fork down and talk to my niece. My sister-in-law urges everyone to have seconds. I smile and tell her I'm still enjoying my firsts.

either fail to lose or wind up regaining. It simply isn't true! We now know that this pessimistic prognosis is based mainly on the atypical experience of patients in hospital-based programmes. But many people manage to lose weight and keep it off with little or no medical assistance. You probably have lots of friends and relatives who have succeeded. Remember the National Weight Control Registry, which I mentioned in Chapter 2? When scientists from the University of Pittsburgh announced that they wanted to gather information on successful dieters, they had no problem finding hundreds of volunteers.

No matter what has happened before, you can lose weight now. Don't be discouraged by earlier efforts. Research on ex-smokers indicates that it takes four or five tries to end up quitting for good. Ninety-one per cent of the Weight Control Registry members had tried to lose numerous times before the attempt that finally worked. They eventually succeeded—and you can too.

SECRET #2: TAKE RESPONSIBILITY

I've just urged you to believe that weight loss is possible. Now I want to acknowledge that it definitely is not easy. You may be fighting a sluggish metabolism. You may have a full schedule that leaves no obvious time for exercise. And it's tough to modify lifelong eating habits. Food, unlike smoking, is not something you can just give up. Also, eating isn't merely a biological function; it's part of our social and emotional lives. These are real difficulties, and you deserve lots of credit for resolving to surmount them.

Experts—doctors, dietitians, trainers, therapists—can offer assistance, as I'll discuss in Chapter 6; friends and family members can provide support. All this is very valuable. But some people look to others for more than just information and encouragement; they're hoping for someone else to *take responsibility*. For instance, a woman may ask her doctor to weigh her every week; or she might tell her husband, "Please stop me if you see me having seconds." This works for a while—but then her doctor goes on vacation, and she overeats because she doesn't have to worry about her weekly weigh-in. Or she negotiates with her husband for "permission" to have an extra dessert. If she doesn't lose weight, she's not only disappointed for herself, she also feels guilty for letting down the people who are trying to help her—and that's not productive either.

Lean on others at the beginning if you have to, but think of them as the

SOMEONE I LOVE NEEDS TO LOSE WEIGHT— WHAT CAN I DO TO HELP?

♦ Your husband—whose father died young of heart disease— is overweight and sedentary.

♦ Your teenage daughter comes home from school in tears because her classmates call her "The Blimp".

♦ Your best friend hasn't been able to shake her postpartum depression—and you suspect it's because she's still carrying most of the weight she gained during pregnancy.

It's so hard to see a loved one suffer, and so tempting to try to take charge. Sometimes the other person actually begs you for this kind of assistance. Offer your support—but let them assume responsibility. This expression of confidence is the best way to boost their self-esteem.

♦ **Do** help them plan. **Don't** tell them what to do.

♦ **Do** point them to professional help sources if they ask. **Don't** play therapist or dietitian.

♦ **Do** plan nutritious meals; keep wholesome foods on hand for snacks and discard the tempting junk. **Don't** tell them what to eat or what not to eat.

♦ **Do** join them for active sports and exercise sessions. **Don't** become a workout cop.

♦ **Do** praise their successes. **Don't** criticise them when they slip.

equivalent of training wheels on a bicycle: if you continue to depend on their help, you won't go very far. It's fine to ask a friend to join you for your first few aerobic exercise sessions—but don't skip a workout just because she's not available. The people who succeed at weight loss are the ones who take it upon themselves to change their behaviour.

◆ ◆ ◆

My age—44—was sneaking up on me. I felt halfway to 80. I had always been active, but in the last ten years I'd slowed down. I wasn't having fun. Emotionally, I felt I didn't have my life any- more. The only one who could do anything about it was me. I'd been teaching my daughter responsibility. Finally, I told myself to wake up.
—Dianne

◆ ◆ ◆

SECRET #3: SET REALISTIC GOALS

Success provides potent encouragement, even if the achievement is small. So ensure success by setting realistic goals for weight loss.

When I work with a woman who wants to lose weight, one of the first questions I ask her is, "How much do you want to weigh?" It's cause for concern if she gives me a number that's clearly lower than nature intended her to be, a weight that she's never been able to maintain in her entire adult life. When you read Chapter 6, where I discuss weight goals in more detail, you may learn that a healthy weight for you is higher than you thought.

Some people want to drop three dress sizes in eight weeks, or they expect to stick to a very restrictive diet without ever slipping. They may be partly successful, but that's not good enough. So they fail (or think they have failed), get discouraged, and quit. I recently read a 1997 study from the Univer- sity of Pennsylvania with a finding that really frustrated me. Investigators recruited 60 significantly overweight women (their average weight was 98 kilo- grams/ 215 lb) to participate in a 48-week programme. Over the 48 weeks, they lost an average of 16 kilograms (35 lb), a kilo (2 lb) every three weeks. That's a terrific accomplishment! These women should have been thrilled—but many were disappointed. How come? They'd hoped to lose a lot more.

By coincidence, on the same day I saw that report, I read a delightful message from Nancy, a member of the group that tested the programme in this book. Like the women in the University of Pennsylvania study, Nancy has lost about one kilo every three weeks. But what a difference in her attitude:

> *Good news: I have lost another 1.4 kilos (3 lb) to make a total of 8.6 kilos (19 lb) in the past six months. I've also been running/walking 3 kilometres (1.8 miles) almost every day. At first I could only run about a third of the distance, and walked the rest. Now I can run for about three-quarters of it. And yesterday, though I really didn't have the time, I jumped into the swimming pool afterwards and swam three laps. I feel wonderful and full of energy!*

I find that the women most likely to succeed in losing weight are the ones whose chief motivation is to become healthier. They measure their progress not only on the scales but also against fitness goals. Of course, they're pleased to look better; however, they consider this a happy extra. Women whose aim is to fit into a bikini often wind up frustrated by slow weight loss, because they feel they've achieved nothing until they reach their goal. There's a risk they'll push themselves too hard—exercise excessively, restrict their eating too much—and burn out.

I've been discussing your long-term aims, but intermediate goals are important too. It can be overwhelming to look ahead to everything you want to accomplish. If you focus instead on smaller weekly aims, they seem do-able. Achieving these goals is very reinforcing, and makes the next week much easier. Nancy told me:

> *I play games with myself. It's a challenge to see how far I can run. I used to have to stop twice between my house and a particular road. Now I can run all the way, and that makes me feel good.*

Weight loss should be a very positive experience. You're doing something important for yourself—not only becoming slimmer, but also gaining all the benefits of exercise and good nutrition. These improvements happen quickly, even with slow, sensible weight loss. If you enjoy them, you'll reap the rewards of this programme much sooner, and your enthusiasm will remain high.

♦ ♦ ♦

I've lost 26 kilos (57 lb) over an 18-month period, and still have a long way to go. But this is not like waiting for a package to be delivered, where you have nothing until it finally arrives. Yes, I'm still overweight—but I'm already stronger, and I have much more stamina and flexibility. No, I'm not slender. But I look better, and I fit into clothes I haven't been able to wear for years.
        —Jane

♦ ♦ ♦

SECRET #4: MAKE A FIRM COMMITMENT NOW

Think how you make a holiday happen. You don't wait for a time when your schedule is completely empty for two weeks. If you did that, you'd never get a holiday. Instead you pick the dates and make reservations. Suddenly the trip fits into your life—because you make it fit. You switch appointments to clear your calendar; you let friends and colleagues know that you'll be out of town; you arrange for a neighbour to feed the cats and pick up the mail. Pretty soon you're on your way.

You've already taken an important first step towards losing weight: you're reading this book. The second step is to make the decision to follow the programme. Some people get stuck at this point:

I definitely want to try it.
Maybe I'll begin after the holidays.
I'll ask my sister if she wants to do it with me.
One of these days I'll be ready.

Procrastination has insidious effects. Your enthusiasm cools off; your motivation dissolves. You begin to feel guilty about the delay, so you avoid thinking about plans. It becomes increasingly difficult to overcome the inertia.

I urge you to take advantage of your current interest. Assume that you *will* begin strength training and aerobic exercise, that you *will* follow the food plan. Then begin to act on that assumption. Follow the step-by-step instructions in Chapter 10. Obtain the weights, select an aerobic activity, plan menus, and stock up on wholesome foods. Then your healthy new lifestyle will begin.

SECRET #5: PLAN FOR SUCCESS

My schedule is normally very hectic. In addition to a demanding job, I have a husband and three young children. Usually I find the pressure stimulating. But a couple of months ago I took on a few new obligations, then found myself getting frazzled. My tension level increased and my productivity sank.

When I realised what was happening, I made time to sit down and get organised. This made all the difference. As soon as I wrote down my obligations, they stopped crashing around in my head causing friction. I divided big jobs into small, do-able pieces. Tasks that had seemed enormous suddenly shrank. I went through my calendar and figured out when everything would get done. This planning session took about fifteen minutes, but my increased efficiency gave me many hours—and dramatically reduced my stress.

You're about to create significant changes in your life. You'll make decisions about food and exercise; you'll buy equipment and supplies. There will be new skills to learn and new activities to fit into your schedule. That's a lot to tackle at once, even with help from this book. Planning will help you sort everything out so the pieces fall into place. Once you get going, planning will help you continue.

Barbara—a working mother with five children—describes how she set up a weekly routine for exercise:

> *The best time for me to swim is late afternoon, before dinner, when I'm sluggish. I swim on Sundays, Mondays, and Thursdays between four and six o'clock. I try to avoid scheduling parent–teacher meetings or work appointments at those times,*

but if it can't be helped, I substitute a Tuesday swim. This way, I'm never afraid of finding out on Saturday that a week has gone by and I haven't exercised.

Built-in flexibility is an important part of Barbara's plan. It wouldn't work if she couldn't adapt to unexpected demands on her time.

Planning is more than a management strategy; it's a way of nurturing yourself, as Sarah points out:

This may sound trivial, but one of the nicest things I do for myself is to prepare fruit. I cut up a melon after a meal, when I'm not hungry—and later, when I need an instant snack, there it is. I peel and section an orange in the evening—and as if by magic, a ready-to-eat orange is waiting for me in the morning, when I'm still half asleep. If I ever win the lottery, I'm hiring a personal chef. But in the meantime, I can pamper myself this way.

SECRET #6: KEEP RECORDS

Kaiser Permanente, one of America's largest Health Management Organisations, was running a weight-loss programme with over two thousand participants, and the programme leaders wanted to learn what factors were associated with success. They looked at age, activity level, starting weight, and many other variables. What was the best predictor of success? The answer may surprise you: keeping food records. Other studies have corroborated this finding. Indeed, research has shown that people who simply keep food records lose weight, even when they don't consciously eat less. Similar research has found the same for exercise: people who keep logs stick with their exercise programmes.

What makes records so effective? We don't know for sure, but here are some possibilities:

- ♦ Record-keeping reflects characteristics that make for success: strong motivation; attention to programme requirements.

◆ Records help you follow a food or exercise plan, because they keep track of details. For instance, if you tally the day's food allotment, you'll know whether you're eating enough fruit, or if you can take an extra snack without going over. When you write down the dumbbells you lift for each exercise, you know which ones to use the next time. This makes your workouts more efficient.

◆ Records are a constant reminder of your commitment. I often hear comments like this: *I was tempted to take seconds, but I resisted because I didn't want to write it down.*

◆ Over time, records help you see how far you've come. That's very motivating. If you've been sedentary, you may struggle during your first 10-minute aerobics session. Write that down—and read it in a month or two, when you're able to sustain 20 or 30 minutes.

You might think that it takes complicated records to be effective. Not so. Simply checking off boxes on a form makes a big difference. Some people actually like to keep detailed food or exercise logs. They write down exactly what they eat at every meal or snack, and they have similar descriptions of their workouts. That's fine, but most women prefer minimal record keeping.

Members of the group that tested the programme in this book recognised the benefit of recording their workouts. They soon discovered that if they didn't write down the weights they lifted for the arm exercises, they'd forget at least one of them by the next session. Some also took to food logs; but others were considerably less enthusiastic, even though I pointed out that the forms required less than two minutes a day.

I told them: "Some people can stay on track without food records, and it's fine for them to skip this step. However, if you find that you're not doing as well with the food plan as you'd hoped, I urge you to give record keeping a try—you'll be amazed at how potent it is."

SECRET #7: REBOUND— AND LEARN—FROM MISTAKES

If you watch the Olympics, you've seen dramas like this: a figure skater is per-forming a complex programme, the culmination of years of training. She stumbles badly in her first jump, losing points. But despite this confidence-shaking disappointment, she completes the rest of her routine flawlessly and wins.

Learning how to bounce back and persevere is one of the most helpful lessons I've learned from sports psychology, and it's invaluable for many aspects of life, including weight loss. Setbacks are inevitable in any long-term effort. Yet some people become so distracted and demoralised by small failures that they forget their larger successes and go off track. As a result, a problem that should have been small and temporary becomes large and persistent. Remember the University of Maryland study I mentioned earlier, the one that found people who believed in themselves were more successful at weight loss? I think it's significant that the believers were not only more self-confident, they were also less likely than the disbelievers to berate themselves for mistakes—showing the power of the language you use with yourself.

If you overeat at Christmas, you might gain half a kilo (1 lb) or so. That's of little long-term consequence, provided you return to your food plan right away. Here's what sports psychologists tell athletes—I think it's great advice for everyone:

- Don't be self-critical just because you've made an error. Mistakes are unfortunate, but they're a normal part of life. That's why many pencils come with built-in erasers.

- Look back only to learn from what happened, not to criticise yourself. After you've extracted the lessons, move on.

- Concentrate on the task ahead.

- Remind yourself how far you've come toward your long-term goals. You've got a lot to be proud of!

WHAT HAVE YOU GOT

TO LOSE?

*When you're a teenager, you learn all these rules from your girl-
friends: if you stand with your knees touching, there should be a
space between your thighs. Your waist should be 10 inches smaller
than your hips and chest. You should weigh 100 pounds plus five
pounds for each inch over five feet. Even though you grow up and
realise how dumb these rules are, they remain stuck somewhere in
your brain.*

　　　—Alexandra

◆　◆　◆

As you begin this programme and set goals for yourself, you're probably
wondering how much you should weigh. That's a very good question,
but I can't provide a simple answer. I'll start by giving you the same
suggestion I give to the women I work with: if you have a particular weight in
mind, set it aside for a moment so you can take a fresh look. What's important
really isn't a specific number on a scale, but looking good, being healthy,
and feeling vibrant and fit. Moreover, your aims need to be tempered with

realism. If you try to become thinner than you've ever been in your adult life, you'll have to struggle to achieve and maintain the lower weight.

In addition to thinking about your goals, you'll need to decide whether you should see a doctor or arrange for other assistance before you begin. This chapter will help you through these preliminaries—and then you'll be ready to start.

◆　　◆　　◆

I have an 11-year-old daughter. I want her to be strong, to exercise, and to eat well, so she'll be confident and feel really good about herself. And I want her to do all these things for healthy reasons, without worrying about what she looks like. So I'm trying to be a good role model for her.
　　—Therese

◆　　◆　　◆

THAT MAGIC NUMBER

When I talk to women about their weight goals, many of them admit that they're still fixed on a number—a weight or a dress size—left over from their teenage years. Because that magic number represents being attractive and slender, it carries a lot of emotional baggage. Jill told me:

I wanted to be like Margot Fonteyn: 167 centimetres (65 in), 56 kilos (123 lb). Today, that would be heavy for a ballet dancer. The trouble was, I reached 167 centimetres (65 in) at age 13 and kept going. But I still remember 56 kilos (123 lb).

Jill agreed to set aside this number and rethink her goals. I asked about her weight history. She is 173 centimetres (67 in) and—except for a period of depression which she gained 9 kilos (20 lb)—her adult weight has been between 64 (141 lb) and 66 (145 lb). Recently the scales have crept into the 66 to 68 (145 to 149 lb) range, which concerns her. Despite the fact that she eats well and does aerobic exercise, her clothes are getting snug.

Many women don't set weight goals when they start this programme. They simply want to get healthier and fitter—and that's absolutely fine. But others, like Jill, want a specific objective. If that's your preference, I believe that three factors are important in coming up with your goal.

- **What's healthy** should be your primary concern—feeling good physically and emotionally. Later in this chapter I'll explain how to determine a healthy weight range for your height. Jill was surprised to learn how wide this range is—in her case, 56 to 74 kilograms (123 to 163 lb). She knew that she'd felt sluggish, bloated, and unattractive during the brief period that she weighed 74 kilograms (163 lb), so that was not a good weight for her.

- **What's realistic** must be carefully considered too. The best indicator is your own history. True, 57 kilograms (125 lb) wouldn't be an unhealthy weight for Jill, but is it realistic? Her normal eating and exercise habits—which had kept her at 64 to 66 kilos (141 to 145 lb) for years—would need to be changed significantly. A woman whose weight or sedentary lifestyle put her at risk of serious health problems has compelling reasons to make major changes. But that wasn't true for Jill.

- **What it takes to look your best** is important—but this is not simply a matter of what you weigh. When you eat well and become fit, you naturally look better. Strength training trims and tightens, so you're slimmer even if you don't shed a kilo. After a few weeks of nutritious eating and good hydration, women whose diet had been haphazard often notice improvements in their appearance: their skin is no longer dry; their hair becomes glossy. Increased self-confidence and energy also do wonders for a person's looks.

A woman who is overweight and unhappy about her appearance sometimes feels that losing weight is the only answer. But there's so much more she can do to look better. I'm sure you've seen makeovers in magazines and on TV, with startlingly different "before" and "after" pictures. The woman is transformed not so much because she has lost weight, but because she has a new haircut, touches of makeup, new glasses, and well-chosen clothes—not to mention that she's smiling happily and standing tall.

Jill realised that her previously normal weight range, 64 to 66 kilograms (141 to 145 lb), was probably best for her. By slightly increasing her aerobic activity and cutting back a little on snacks, she should be able to get there in about 10 weeks. Because she's started strength training, I won't be surprised if she's a size smaller this time than she previously was at that weight. As you read through this chapter, I hope you'll rethink your goals. Most women tell me they feel liberated and unencumbered when they're finally able to unload the unrealistic and burdensome numbers they've carried for years.

♦　♦　♦

A woman in my weight-loss class said that her ideal weight was based on a Barbie doll she had when she was a girl. It came with some scales. Barbie was supposed to be 175 centimetres (65 inches) and the number painted on the scales was 50 kilos (110 lb). That brought home to me the unrealistic goals that people set for themselves.
—Isabel

♦　♦　♦

WHAT'S THE BEST WEIGHT FOR YOUR HEALTH?

In the United States we used to have quaint old scales where you put in a penny and got your weight and fortune. Printed on top was the Metropolitan Life Insurance Company's table of ideal body weights for men and women, by height. Metropolitan Life had gathered data about their customers for decades, and the tables represented what they'd learned about the optimal weights for longevity and health. Their height–weight tables were widely used—most people had seen them in books and magazines or at their doctor's rooms—but they simply created two categories: ideal and everything else. Obviously, the degree of excess weight matters too. So, these days, experts use the Body Mass Index (BMI) instead of the Metropolitan Life tables. The BMI is also the index used in Britain. The underlying information, which comes from insurance company statistics and large-scale health studies, is really the same. However, the BMI combines height and weight into a single number—the higher above normal it is, the greater the health risks.

Body Mass Index (For Women and Men)

1. Read down the first column to locate your height.
2. Read across that row and locate your weight.
3. Read the heading on top of the column—that's your BMI.

Height (cm)	18 or less	19	20	21	22	23	24	25	26	27	28	29	30	31	32	33	34	35	36
148	39	41	43	45	47	50	52	54	56	58	61	62	65	67	69	71	73	75	78
150	40	43	45	47	49	51	53	56	58	60	62	65	67	69	71	74	74	78	81
152	42	44	46	48	51	53	55	58	60	62	65	67	69	71	74	76	79	81	83
154	43	45	48	50	52	55	57	60	62	65	67	69	71	74	76	79	81	84	86
156	44	47	49	52	54	56	59	61	64	66	69	71	74	76	78	81	84	86	89
158	46	48	51	53	56	59	61	64	66	69	71	74	76	78	81	84	87	89	91
160	47	50	52	55	58	61	63	65	68	71	74	76	79	81	84	87	89	94	95
162	49	51	54	57	59	62	65	68	71	73	76	79	81	84	87	89	92	95	98
164	50	53	56	59	61	64	67	70	73	75	78	81	84	87	90	92	95	98	101
166	52	55	57	61	63	66	69	72	75	78	81	84	86	89	92	95	98	101	104
168	53	56	59	62	65	68	71	74	77	80	83	86	89	92	95	98	101	104	107
170	55	58	61	64	67	70	73	76	80	82	86	89	92	95	98	101	104	107	110
172	56	59	63	66	69	72	75	79	82	85	88	91	95	98	101	104	107	110	113
174	58	61	65	68	71	75	78	81	84	87	91	94	97	100	104	107	110	113	117
176	59	63	66	70	73	76	80	83	86	90	93	96	100	103	106	110	113	117	120

BMI under 19: Underweight
BMI 19 to 25: Healthy weight
BMI 26 to 30: Overweight
BMI 31 to 39: Very overweight
BMI 40 and above: Extremely overweight

HOW TO CALCULATE YOUR BMI

Here's a three-step method for computing your BMI if you know your weight and height. A calculator will help.

Step 1: Multiply your weight in pounds by 703.

Step 2: Multiply your height in inches by itself.

Step 3: Divide the first number by the second.

Round to the nearest whole number—that's your BMI.
Example: Gretchen weighs 180 pounds; she's 5 feet, 5 inches tall.

Step 1: $180 \times 703 = 126{,}540$

Step 2: $65 \times 65 = 4{,}225$

Step 3: $126{,}540 \div 4{,}225 = 29.95$ So Gretchen's BMI is 30.

The web site of Shape Up America —a superb fitness and nutrition program initiated by former US Surgeon General Dr C. Everett Koop—has BMI tables and information. If you provide your height and weight, you can learn your BMI instantly. The URL is: http://www.shapeup.org.

THE BODY MASS INDEX

Your BMI is your weight in kilograms divided by the square of your height in metres—but don't sharpen your pencil yet! The simplest way to determine your BMI is to look it up on a chart (see page 91); or you can use the instructions on this page to do the calculation in pounds and inches.

WHAT'S YOUR BMI?

If you've recently had your weight and height measured on a medical visit, use those numbers. Otherwise follow these procedures. If possible, weigh yourself in the morning, before you eat breakfast. Since the charts are based on weights without clothing, wear as little as possible.

Next, measure your height. You can do this yourself, but it's easier if someone helps you. Stand in bare feet with your back to a wall. Your heels should be against the wall; your head should be held high but not tilted back.

Rest a ruler flat on top of your head, keeping it parallel to the floor. Mark the spot where the ruler touches the wall. Then measure the wall from floor to mark to determine your height.

If you're over the age of 40, it's a good idea to measure your height at least once a year. Getting shorter could be a sign of osteoporosis. If you discover that you've shrunk more than a couple of centimetres (anything less could simply reflect a measurement error), tell your doctor.

The Body Mass Index chart is on page 91. First, find your number, then read through what it means.

How to Interpret Your BMI

Your BMI tells you whether your weight falls into a range that's optimal for longevity and good health. However, I want to emphasise that you're an individual, not a statistic. Weight, though important, is just one factor in determining your risk of disease; lifestyle, family history, and current health also matter. For instance, if you're overweight but fit and healthy, you're at much lower risk of heart disease than someone who has the same BMI or even lower but who is sedentary and suffering from diabetes.

BMI Under 19: Underweight

Because excess weight is such a prevalent problem, we sometimes forget that it's not healthy to be underweight either. A BMI under 19 is associated with elevated risk of cancer; osteoporosis; and infertility; and emotional problems, including anxiety, depression, suicide, and sleep difficulties. Since emotional problems may be tied to eating disorders, which can be life-threatening, it's very important to seek diagnosis and appropriate treatment. (See box on eating disorders on page 94.)

If your BMI is below 19, you should not attempt to lose weight. However, you can use the *Strong Women Stay Slim* programme to become fitter and to develop healthier eating patterns. I often see women who are underweight but over-fat—they're thin but not toned. If your body is like that, you certainly don't need to lose weight. Strengthening exercise and aerobics will make you stronger, firmer and shapelier.

BMI Between 19 and 25: Healthy Weight

This BMI range is associated with the longest life and lowest risk for disease. The range is wider than you might expect, because it covers men as well as women, and people of all ages and different builds. I realise that some

MIGHT YOU HAVE AN EATING DISORDER?

Women with eating disorders come in all different sizes, from thin to heavy. The following statements are adapted from material developed by the USA organisation Anorexia Nervosa and Related Eating Disorders, Inc. The more numerous the items that apply to you, the more serious your problem may be—and the more important it is for you to seek help.

- Even though my doctor and my friends tell me I'm thin, I feel fat.

- Other people worry about the way I eat; I lie about my eating.

- When I eat, I'm afraid I won't be able to stop.

- I feel guilty when I eat.

- I have missed work or school because of my weight or eating habits.

- When I eat, I feel bloated and fat.

- I do strange things with my food—for example, cut it into tiny pieces, eat it on special dishes with special utensils, make patterns on my plate with it, secretly spit it out.

- To control my weight, I vomit, take laxatives or diuretics, or fast.

- I get anxious if I can't exercise.

- I have said or thought, "I would rather die than be fat."

- I have noticed one or more of the following: irregular or absent menstrual periods (even though I'm premenopausal), cold hands and feet, dry skin, thinning hair, fragile nails, swollen glands in my neck, dental cavities, dizziness, weakness, fainting, rapid or irregular heartbeat.

For referrals and further information about eating disorders:

EATING DISORDERS ASSOCIATION
First Floor, Wensum House
103 Prince of Wales Road
Norwich
Norfolk NR1 1DW
Tel: 01603 621414 (HELPLINE)

INTERNATIONAL EATING DISORDERS CENTRE
119/121 Wendover Road
Aylesbury
Buckinghamshire HP21 9LW
Tel: 01296 330557

OVEREATERS ANONYMOUS
PO Box 19
Stretford
Manchester M32 9EB
Tel: 01426 984674

ANOREXIA ANONYMOUS
24 Westmoreland Road
Barnes
London SW13
Tel: 0181 878 9199

women in this category are not happy with their weight—they don't feel "ideal" at all—while others are perfectly content.

What's a reasonable goal for you? Ask yourself these questions:

◆ **Are you at above-average risk of heart disease or diabetes?** If so, I'd suggest you aim for a BMI at the mid to low end of the ideal range.

What's Your Waist-to-Hip Ratio?

Excess fat around the abdomen—a high waist-to-hip ratio—is strongly associated with **Syndrome X**, a cluster of symptoms that signal elevated risk of both heart disease and diabetes: high blood pressure, resistance to insulin, and high levels of cholesterol and other fat in the blood. This is why doctors are more concerned when an overweight person has a large belly rather than big hips and thighs.

Are you at risk for Syndrome X? To find out, first measure your waist. Some people have an obvious waistline. If yours isn't clear, find the smallest circumference between the upper part of your hipbone and the lowest part of your rib cage on your side, and measure that. The tape should be neither tight nor loose. Women are at elevated risk if their waist is 90 centimetres (35 inches) or larger.

If your waist is less than 90 centimetres (35 inches), you'll need to calculate your waist-to-hip ratio to assess your risk. Measure the widest point on your hips. Then divide your waist measurement by your hip measurement.

- **Favourable**: Waist-to-hip ratio less than .8

- **Borderline**: Waist-to-hip ratio between .8 and .85

- **Unfavourable**: Waist-to-hip ratio above .85, or waist 90 centimetres (35 inches) or larger

Though there's a strong genetic component to body shape, aerobic exercise and weight loss can decrease waist size and the waist-to-hip ratio.

- **What's your weight history?** If you know you feel and look better at the mid to low end of the ideal range, that's a good goal. However, I don't recommend you aim for a weight you've never been able to sustain. Instead, concentrate on going down one or two BMI points, while eating well and becoming fit. At that point, if you're still not satisfied, you can always lose some more.

♦ **Are you unhappy about your appearance?** As you start to eat better and exercise more, you will undoubtedly see improvements—and possibly a difference on the scales as well. Most women who follow this programme find that they're satisfied with themselves at a heavier weight than they would have expected. Because muscle is more compact than fat, they become smaller even if their weight doesn't drop. Also, they have a more positive body image, greater self-esteem, and increased vitality—and that makes a big difference.

BMI Between 26 and 30: Moderately Overweight
BMI Between 31 and 39: Very Overweight
BMI 40 and up: Extremely Overweight

The higher your BMI, the greater the risk that you'll suffer from weight-related disability or disease. Individuals with a BMI of 40 and over are at substantial risk. The danger is further increased if you have a high waist-to-hip ratio (see box) and additional risk factors, such as high blood pressure or elevated blood cholesterol or blood sugar.

If you are in any of these three BMI categories, I suggest that you set as an initial goal losing enough weight to move down two BMI numbers. This change has been shown to improve health, especially if accomplished with increased physical activity and improved nutrition. If you have any of the additional risk factors mentioned above, you should see an effect on them too. As a longer-term goal, try to bring yourself down to the next lower BMI category. If you're already suffering from weight-related illness or disability, the change will probably make a big difference in your symptoms.

Don't be discouraged if you have a long way to go. You'll see significant improvements very quickly, even if you're still overweight. As you progress, you'll feel and look better. And with each lower BMI number, your health risks are reduced. Think of two BMI numbers as a stepping-stone, and focus on moving down just one step at a time.

Physical Activity Readiness
Questionnaire—PAR-Q
(revised 1994)

PAR-Q & YOU

(A Questionnaire for People Aged 15 to 69)

Regular physical activity is fun and healthy, and increasingly more people are starting to become more active every day. Being more active is very safe for most people. However, some people should check with their doctor before they start becoming much more physically active.

If you are planning to become much more physically active than you are now, start by answering the seven questions in the box below. If you are between the ages of 15 and 69, the PAR-Q will tell you if you should check with your doctor before you start. If you are over 69 years of age, and you are not used to being very active, check with your doctor.

Common sense is your best guide when you answer these questions. Please read the questions carefully and answer each one honestly: check YES or NO.

YES NO

☐ ☐ 1. Has your doctor ever said that you have a heart condition <u>and</u> that you should only do physical activity recommended by a doctor?

☐ ☐ 2. Do you feel pain in your chest when you do physical activity?

☐ ☐ 3. In the past month, have you had chest pain when you were not doing physical activity?

☐ ☐ 4. Do you lose your balance because of dizziness or do you ever lose consciousness?

☐ ☐ 5. Do you have a bone or joint problem that could be made worse by a change in your physical activity?

☐ ☐ 6. Is your doctor currently prescribing drugs (for example, water pills) for your blood pressure or heart condition?

☐ ☐ 7. Do you know of <u>any other reason</u> why you should not do physical activity?

IF **YOU ANSWERED**

YES to one or more questions

Talk with your doctor by phone or in person BEFORE you start becoming much more physically active or BEFORE you have a fitness appraisal. Tell your doctor about the PAR-Q and which questions you answered YES.

- ♦ You may be able to do any activity you want—as long as you start slowly and build up gradually. Or, you may need to restrict your activities to those which are safe for you. Talk with your doctor about the kinds of physical activities you wish to participate in and follow his/her advice.
- ♦ Find out which community programs are safe and helpful for you.

NO to all questions

If you answered NO honestly to *all* PAR-Q questions, you can be reasonably sure that you can:

- ♦ start becoming much more physically active—begin slowly and build up gradually. This is the safest and easiest way to go.
- ♦ take part in a fitness appraisal—this is an excellent way to determine your basic fitness so that you can plan the best way for you to live actively.

DELAY BECOMING MUCH MORE ACTIVE:

- ♦ if you are not feeling well because of a temporary illness such as a cold or fever—wait until you feel better; or
- ♦ if you are or may be pregnant—talk to your doctor before you start becoming more active.

Please note: If your health changes so that you then answer YES to any of the above questions, tell your fitness or health professional. Ask whether you should change your physical activity plan.

DO YOU NEED TO SEE YOUR DOCTOR?

Many women skip medical check-ups. They're busy; they're feeling fine and don't see the need; they worry about the expense or fear bad news. If you haven't had a check-up for a year or more, please make an appointment. Routine physical examinations can detect cancer and other serious medical problems long before symptoms appear, when treatment is most effective.

Overweight women may avoid the doctor out of embarrassment, or because they expect criticism. If such concerns have held you back in the past, I hope you feel more confident now that you're starting this programme. A supportive doctor will discuss diet and exercise strategies, and take baseline measurements—such as weight, blood pressure, blood cholesterol, and blood sugar—that will help you track your progress. If your doctor isn't helpful, don't be shy about expressing your concern and asking for what you need. If you aren't satisfied with the response, consider seeking another physician.

BEFORE YOU TRY TO LOSE WEIGHT

Your doctor may have already told you that losing weight is not only safe but also highly desirable. However, some women have physical conditions that make weight loss inappropriate, even if they're currently overweight. For example, losing weight is not advised during pregnancy. If you have any progressive medical condition—including Parkinson's, multiple sclerosis, or rheumatoid arthritis—discuss your weight goals with your doctor before starting this programme.

BEFORE YOU CHANGE YOUR DIET

The food plan in this programme follows well-established nutrition guidelines for healthy women. However, some individuals will need to modify it. Discuss the diet with your doctor if you're pregnant or breast-feeding, or if you follow a therapeutic diet for a medical condition, such as diabetes or kidney disease.

BEFORE YOU BEGIN EXERCISING

The exercise programmes in this book are safe for nearly everyone. However, some women should talk to a doctor before increasing their physical activity. Take the PAR-Q—Physical Activity Readiness Questionnaire—to see if this caution applies to you. Remember, if you're in doubt, err on the side of safety and check with your doctor.

COULD YOU USE SOME EXTRA HELP?

I've tried to make this book as comprehensive as possible, but you may know from past experience that you'll need extra support. Working one-to-one with a professional can make a big difference—and it may not be as costly as you'd expect. Even if you have to bear the cost of professional assistance and are limited in what you can afford, a few sessions could be very valuable, especially when you're getting started or if you run into problems later on.

Useful help sources include dietitians, exercise trainers, psychologists and support groups.

DIETITIANS

My family won't eat "diet food" and I don't have time to cook separate meals.

Menu planning is a problem for me.

When I go on a diet, I'm hungry all the time.

The food plan in this book is a healthy way of eating that will benefit every member of your family. But they may take a little convincing—I'll have some suggestions about that in Chapter 11. A dietitian could help you devise menus that match your family's preferences (and yours).

The initials SRD, which stand for State Registered Dietitian, mean that a dietician has met the stringent requirements of the the British Dietetic Association. To find an SRD in your area, ask your doctor or contact the British Dietetic Association on 0121 643 5483.

EXERCISE TRAINERS

I find it hard to follow instructions from a book.
I've got a bad elbow, so I worry about doing some of the exercises.
I'd like some moves to address my "love handles".

Although most people won't need a trainer to learn the exercises in this book, others do better with extra assistance. A trainer can help you learn the moves and proper form for strength-training exercises and aerobic work-outs. As you progress, the trainer can recheck your form, answer questions, and offer encouragement. When you're ready to make changes—such as expanding your strength-training programme or beginning a new kind of aerobic exercise—the trainer can advise you.

Many exercise class instructors see clients privately. Get a referral from a local health club (even if you're not a member), or call an adult education programme. Make sure the trainer has experience working with people like you, especially if you have special concerns or unusual needs. The trainer should be registered with one of the following registration bodies: the National Register of Personal Trainers (0181 944 6688), which maintains a database of qualified, experienced and insured trainers in the UK; the Association of Personal Trainers (0171 836 1102) which is affiliated to the Exercise Association of England.

◆   ◆   ◆

When I began strength training I worked with a trainer because I have a tendency to get hurt. I have chronic back pain from a tennis injury I got more than twenty years ago. The trainer taught me strengthening exercises for my upper and lower body, and also suggested limbering exercises. She told me to stop doing an exercise I was using for back pain—and my back got better. When I had a flare-up, she helped me modify my workouts.
—Judith

◆   ◆   ◆

PSYCHOLOGISTS

My eating is so out of control that it scares me sometimes.

When I lose weight and begin to look different, I become anxious and depressed and I start overeating again.

Other people undermine my efforts if I try to lose weight: my husband complains about the time I spend exercising; my mother says I'm too thin; my best friend says I'm no fun anymore. I don't know how to cope with this.

Sometimes women gain weight because they're going through a troubled period; for other women, eating and weight become so entangled with emotion that change is difficult. Once they get help, it's easier to follow a programme of sensible eating and exercise—and often many other aspects of their lives improve as well.

Consider seeking psychological assistance when you suspect that deeper emotional issues are getting in your way. Try to find a therapist who specialises in weight-related problems. This is especially important if you suspect that you might have an eating disorder. Good referral sources are your doctor, or the psychology, psychiatry, or clinical nutrition department at a local teaching hospital; the organisations listed in the box about eating disorders (page 95) also provide referrals.

SUPPORT GROUPS

I need lots of encouragement, but my family and friends get tired of hearing about my diet.

It really inspires me to see "Before" and "After" pictures of people who've lost weight.

For me, the best advice comes from other women who are doing the same thing.

Weight-loss support groups provide companionship and inspiration, plus a ready source of helpful tips. As you get slimmer and fitter, you'll have the satisfaction of serving as a model for others.

Your doctor can probably refer you to a group. Groups vary, even within the same organisation, so check out others if you don't care for the first one you try. Another option is an online support group.

◆ ◆ ◆

I'm good at networking. I get a lot of support by talking to people and sharing ideas. A core group of people in my diet group showed up every week. What we liked most was talking about strategies—practical, usable stuff: How do you deal with eating at a restaurant? What are your techniques for not eating when something is seducing you? How do you manage at parties?
—Therese

◆ ◆ ◆

If you need more than one kind of help, call a local teaching hospital or community health centre. Many have excellent weight-reduction programmes that offer multiple resources, including doctors, dietitians, exercise physiologists, psychologists, and support groups.

III

THE STRONG WOMEN STAY SLIM PROGRAMME

▼ ▼ ▼ ▼

7

SIX EXERCISES THAT WILL MAKE YOU STRONG

I can run upstairs without my knees killing me for the first time in many years. I'm a professional violinist, and I'm finding that my increased upper body strength has been a real boost to my endurance during long performances—an unexpected bonus! And all of this after only a few weeks of strength training.
— Sue

◆ ◆ ◆

Strength training is the foundation of the *Strong Women Stay Slim* weight-loss programme. The exercise plan outlined in this chapter requires just three 20-minute sessions per week, but it produces extraordinary effects. The major muscle groups in your body—your arms, shoulders, back, abdomen, buttocks, and legs—will become significantly stronger. Strength training is exciting because you notice improvements in a few weeks. That's around the time you begin aerobic activity. And behind the scenes, these exercises build muscle and bone tissue, so your body gets leaner and healthier as you lose weight.

The key to success with strength training is to start at an easy level and work up slowly but steadily. I'll explain exactly how to customise the programme to give you the right challenge. This chapter also includes two extra strengthening exercises that you can incorporate after a month or two, when you're ready for more.

GEAR

To strengthen your muscles, you have to work them harder than usual. Four of the exercises use dumbbells. The others use your own body weight: by changing position, you can increase or decrease the load on your muscles. You don't have to join a gym, buy costly weight machines, or purchase ankle cuffs. All you need are dumbbells and a container or rack to hold them, plus a few simple items you probably have around the house.

DUMBBELLS

During the first week, most women do the exercises with 1.35-kilogram (3-lb) weights. But you'll move up very quickly, and eventually go past 4.5-kg (10-lb) for most of the arm exercises.

While buying a complete set of dumbbells is really best, it's expensive and takes up a lot of space. So here's my suggestion for a workable compromise between convenience and cost:

♦ Instead of starting with 1.35-kilogram (3-lb) dumbbells—which you'll probably use only for the first two weeks—do the exercises holding a 1-kilogram (2-lb) can of food or fruit juice in each hand. Select tall, narrow cans rather than short, wide ones, so you can hold them securely. Note: I do not recommend using larger cans when you graduate to heavier weights, because they're too big to grip safely.

♦ Buy pairs of dumbbells in 1.35-kg (3-lb), 2.25-kg (5-lb), 3.60-kg (8-lb), 4.50-kg (10-lb) and 6.80-kg (15-lb) weights. Two suggestions for economising: first, check out the sets of dumbbells sold by many sport shops; buying a set and filling in the missing weights may save you money. Second, see if you can skip the 1.35-kilogram weights: start the programme with 1 kilogram cans. Then go to the store and try the lifts with 2.25-kilogram (5-lb) weights. Some women can move directly to 2.25-kilogram (5-lb) dumbbells.

♦ To keep initial costs down, don't buy heavier weights immediately. Wait until you've progressed to 5-kilogram weights on some of the exercises. At that point, women typically need 4.50-kg (10-lb) and 6.80-kg (15-lb) dumbbells to get the most out of the programme.

You can also save money by sharing weights with friends, or buying used dumbbells. For safety's sake, I don't recommend improvising using water jugs or buckets as equipment; these are not designed for strength training and could be unsafe. The small investment required for good equipment makes sense—after all, you're spending your valuable time on these workouts.

Dumbbells up to 4.50 kg (10 lb) are sold in discount and department stores, as well as in shops that sell sporting equipment. However, for heavier dumbbells, you'll probably need a specialty shop. Check the Yellow Pages under "Sports Goods Shops" to find shops near you, and call to make sure they have what you require. Alternatively, you can contact the following specialists who will refer you to your closest retail outlet:

BODYPOWER SPORTS
2a Allen Road
Northampton NN1 4NE
Tel: 01604 603248
Fax: 01604 26966

THE PHYSICAL COMPANY
Cherry Cottage
Bourne End
Buckinghamshire SL8 5DH
Tel: 01628 520208
Fax: 01628 851249

CONTAINER FOR THE WEIGHTS

Always keep your dumbbells in a sturdy container or on a rack when you're not actually lifting them. Possibilities include a strong canvas tote bag or duffel bag (the handles are convenient) or a sturdy box.

CHAIR

You'll do some of the exercises while seated in a chair, and for other moves you'll stand and hold the back of the chair for balance. Select a chair that's sturdy, with a seat sufficiently high and deep so that when you sit back in it your knee joint is just over the edge. To allow for free movement, the chair should be armless. Also, be sure the back is high enough to hold on to without leaning over.

CLOTHING

You don't need special clothes for strength training—which is very handy if you do the exercises during a break at work. Clothing needs to be sufficiently loose so you can move freely, and breathable so you don't get hot. Trainers or athletic shoes are best; other low-heel shoes are acceptable, so long as they're flexible and sturdy.

WHAT ABOUT OTHER TYPES OF STRENGTH-TRAINING EQUIPMENT?

Women sometimes ask me about exercise elastic bands, because they're light and inexpensive. Though bands can be very beneficial, and even if these are available where you live, it's difficult to follow a progressive programme with them, and they can be cumbersome to use correctly. Therefore, I prefer dumbbells.

Strength-training machines—both at-home and gym versions—can give you a terrific workout. To follow the *Strong Women Stay Slim* programme with machines, just make sure you target the same muscle groups (a trainer can help). The same basic principles apply.

GENERAL INSTRUCTIONS FOR STRENGTH TRAINING

Strength training is safe for nearly everyone—especially if you heed the simple precautions below, which also make for more effective workouts.

CREATE A SAFE EXERCISE AREA

Clear a space for training that's large enough for your chair plus dumbbells. If possible, place the chair on a secure carpet, so it doesn't slide. If your floors are bare, stabilise the chair by putting it against a wall.

BACK SAFETY TIPS

Caution: if you've ever had back problems, or if you have osteoporosis, discuss this programme with your doctor before you begin.

The following tips are for everyone—but pay special attention if you need to pamper your back:

- Be just as careful when moving weights to and from the workout area as you are when you do the exercises.
- If possible, store your dumbbells next to your workout area, so you don't have to move them for each session.
- Lift the container properly: bend at the knees and rise slowly.

Store your dumbbells in a container when you're not using them. As soon as you finish an exercise, put away the weights. Never leave dumbbells on a table or a shelf—it's all too easy for them to roll off and drop on a foot. **Keep weights safely away from children and pets.**

♦ ♦ ♦

Even my 6-year-old niece has noticed that I'm strong. The other day she said to me: "Mummy can't pick me up anymore, but you can. I know why—it's because you lift weights."
—*Susan*

♦ ♦ ♦

MAINTAIN GOOD POSTURE

Proper posture helps avoid muscle strain and injury when you strength train—but that's just one of its benefits. Standing tall is the fastest way to look pounds lighter and years younger. As your back and abdominal muscles get stronger, good posture becomes easier and easier.

Whether you're sitting or standing, your body should be relaxed but straight, as if someone had fastened a string to the top of your head and was pulling you up. Check yourself in a mirror, or ask a friend to check you.

PERFORM THE LIFTS SLOWLY

Most of us, unless we watch ourselves, tend to perform the lifts too quickly or to speed up as a session continues. For safety and for best results, it's important to do the exercises slowly. If you simply swing the weight or drop it, you could injure your back or shoulders. What's more, your muscles won't become trained if momentum or gravity does the work.

COUNT OUT LOUD WHILE YOU EXERCISE

Counting aloud reminds you to move slowly. Also, it ensures proper breathing; if you're counting you're not likely to hold your breath—a common mistake.

Good posture

- Chin is tipped in, so it's in line with the neck.

- Neck is in line with the spine.

- Shoulders are back, down, and relaxed.

- Back is straight.

- Pelvis is slightly tucked under.

- Knees are neither locked nor bent.

PROGRESS AT THE RECOMMENDED PACE

Some women become so enthusiastic about strength training that they press forward prematurely and attempt to lift weights that are too heavy. Try to be patient. If you advance too soon, you'll find it hard to maintain proper form and you could hurt yourself. Your tendons and ligaments, which generally aren't as strong as your muscles, need time to catch up. When you progress slowly, everything strengthens together.

It's important to allow at least one day for your muscles to recover between exercise sessions. Strength training creates microscopic tears in muscles, an accelerated version of the normal wear and tear from everyday life. What makes you stronger is the body's repair and rebuilding process, and that takes a little time.

Relax!

In the instructions for each exercise, I'll remind you to check your body for tension—and to relax.

- **Face:** Keep your face relaxed; don't furrow or knit your brow.

- **Jaw and neck:** Avoid clenching your teeth or tightening your jaw. If your jaw is relaxed, your neck will be relaxed too.

- **Shoulders:** Don't scrunch your shoulders up toward your ears. Keep them back and relaxed.

- **Legs and arms:** Only the muscles you're exercising should be tensed. All other muscles in your body should be relaxed. Don't lock your knees.

If you need to stop strength training for two or more weeks, don't expect to resume at the point where you were before. Reduce the amount you lift, or drop back to an easier version of the exercises, just to be on the safe side; you can always increase the weight again as your muscles re-adjust.

♦   ♦   ♦

Every September there's a river clean-up day in my community. Last year I mainly watched. But this year I put waders on and pulled rubbish out of the water. Under a railway bridge there were huge pieces of rails and old train switches. A group of men were there, waiting for other men to help them. I have prematurely white hair, so they probably thought I was someone's grand-mother. I started hauling out these big pieces of rusted metal—15, 20, 22 kilos (33, 44, 48 lb). They were very surprised.
    —Isabel

♦   ♦   ♦

SIX BASIC STRENGTH-TRAINING EXERCISES

The basic programme calls for three 20-minute exercise sessions per week; each session includes six exercises plus a stretch. All exercises use your own weight for resistance. It's a good idea to warm up your muscles to prepare them for a workout. The first exercise in this programme—the chair stand—serves as a warm-up.

In strength training, a complete move is called a **lift** or repetition. In this programme, eight repetitions, or reps, make a **set**, and you do two sets of each exercise. A lift takes about nine seconds: four seconds to raise the weight, a one-second pause, and four seconds to return to the starting position. You'll stop for a few seconds to take a breath between lifts. Rest about one minute between sets. Though it's not necessary, you may want to pause for a minute or two when you finish an exercise before you go on to the next.

You'll start with light weights or the easiest version of the exercise. In the beginning you'll progress rapidly, and within a few weeks you'll be training at the proper intensity: you'll be able to perform each exercise eight times in good form, but this effort should be close to your limit. When the eighth lift is no longer a challenge, it's time to increase the load.

CHAIR STAND

This super exercise tackles several important muscle groups at once. You'll strengthen and tone your thighs, and work your back and abdominal muscles as well as your buttocks. Chair stands also improve your balance. Plus, this exercise is a great warm-up—which is why it comes first.

Start with Version 1, in which you can use your hands to help. When you find the move easy, progress to Version 2—no-hands. Others will find even Version 1 difficult. In that case, you can use your hands to help you rise and sit down again. And in a few weeks you should be able to do it without hands.

Version 1

Starting position

Sit toward the front of the chair seat, with your knees at a 90-degree angle, and your feet flat on the floor and shoulder-width (about 40 to 45 centimetres/15 to 18 inches) apart. Lightly grip the sides of the seat.

The move

- **1-2-3-Up:** Keeping your back straight, lean forward slightly and slowly stand up. If necessary, use your hands to push off.
- **Pause for a breath.**
- **1-2-3-Down:** *Slowly* return to the starting position— if necessary, using your hands to guide you back to the chair.
- **Pause for a breath, then repeat.**

Where you will feel the effort

In your thighs and buttocks.

Sets and reps

Do eight repetitions for one set. Rest for a minute or two and do a second set.

Notes

The key to success with this exercise is to move slowly, especially as you return to the chair. Use your leg and buttock muscles to lower yourself—*don't* fall back into the seat.

- Remember to move slowly.
- Lean just slightly forward as you start the move.
- Don't hold your breath.
- Check for tension, and relax.

Version 2: Reverse Chair Stand

This version increases effort in two ways: first, it adds the weight of your outstretched arms; second, it's based on a standing rather than seated position. As a result, your abdominal and lower back muscles have to work harder. Don't attempt to do the Reverse Chair Stand until

Version 1 has become easy for you. Later you can make Version 2 even tougher by lowering yourself almost to the chair, but not actually touching it before you pause and rise again.

▼　▼　▼　▼　▼　▼　▼　▼　▼　▼　▼　▼　▼　▼　▼　▼

Starting position

Sit down in the chair, then stand up; this preliminary assures that you're a safe distance from the chair, and won't land on the floor when you sit during the exercise. Stand in front of the chair with head high, feet shoulder-width apart, toes slightly turned out. Extend both arms straight out in front of you, parallel to the floor, with the palms facing down.

The move

◆ **1-2-3-Sit:** Slowly lower yourself into the chair. Keep your chin up, with your eyes facing forward throughout the move. Bend at your hips, keeping your back straight. Aim your buttocks backwards and lean slightly forwards. Don't let yourself fall into the chair! The pull should come from your muscles, not gravity.

◆ **Pause for a breath.**

◆ **1-2-3-Stand:** Slowly raise yourself back to the starting position.

◆ **Pause for a breath, then repeat.**

Where you will feel the effort

In your thighs, buttocks, and trunks.

Sets and reps

Do eight repetitions for one set. Rest for a minute or two and do a second set.

▼ ▼ ▼ ▼ ▼ ▼ ▼ ▼ ▼ ▼ ▼ ▼ ▼ ▼ ▼ ▼ ▼

Notes

- Remember to move slowly.
- Don't bend so far forward that your knees move in front of your toes; knees should remain above your ankles.
- Don't hold your breath.
- Check for tension, and relax.

◆   ◆   ◆

I once got stuck on a low sofa at a friend's house, and it was so embarrassing—I had to ask her to pull me up. This would never happen now that I've lost weight and strengthened my legs.
—Alexandra

◆   ◆   ◆

Overhead Press

Here's a great exercise for your arms and shoulders. The muscles of the shoulders and the backs of the upper arms are notoriously weak in women. That's why it's so difficult to hoist heavy objects over your head—as you may have discovered if you've ever tried to lift a suitcase into the overhead compartment on an aeroplane. Toning these muscles firms those unwelcome "batwings" on the backs of upper arms, and contributes to good posture. Another bonus: improved flexibility. Suddenly you can reach that back zip!

Starting position

Stand straight with a dumbbell in each hand, feet shoulder-width (about 40 to 45 centimetres/15 to 18 inches) apart. Hold the dumbbells up, parallel to the floor, with the inner ends touching the front sides of your shoulders. Your palms should face forward.

The move

- **1-2-3-Up:** Push the dumbbells straight up from the starting position until your arms are over your head. The dumbbells should be slightly in front of your body when your arms are fully extended.
- **Pause for a breath.**
- **1-2-3-Down:** Slowly lower the dumbbells back to the starting position.
- **Pause for a breath, then repeat.**

Where you will feel the effort

In your upper arms, shoulders, and upper back.

Sets and reps

Do eight repetitions for one set. Rest for a minute or two and do a second set.

Notes

♦ Make sure the dumbbells don't move forward or out to the side as you perform the lift; they should go straight up.

- Maintain good posture; don't scrunch your shoulders or arch your back.

- Move slowly.

- Don't hold your breath.

- Check for tension, and relax.

◆ ◆ ◆

I like the fact that I'm building muscle—it makes me feel like a fuel-burning engine. I like feeling stronger. I think it's really important for women to get strong. You don't feel as dependent; you don't always have to ask your husband for help.
    —Jane

◆ ◆ ◆

Bent-Over Row

Several important muscle groups get a workout from this exercise. You'll train the biceps muscles in front of your upper arms, as well as back and shoulder muscles. Your back and abdominal muscles are challenged too, since they work hard to keep your torso stable. Don't be surprised if people start asking whether you've lost weight—as your upper body gets stronger, you'll automatically stand taller, which makes you look slimmer.

Starting position

Sit forward in the chair with your feet flat on the floor, shoulder-width (40 to 45 centimetres/15 to 18 inches) apart, with a dumbbell in each hand. Let your arms hang down at your sides, palms facing in.

Contract your abdominal muscles to hold your torso stable. Bend slightly forward at the waist, with your back straight, until your chest is just above your thighs. Your arms will move forward slightly until they're just behind your lower legs, parallel to them.

The move

- **1-2-3-Up:** Using your shoulder and upper back muscles, pull both dumbbells straight up, as high as you can. Your shoulder blades should move closer together. Your elbows will need to bend, but most of the effort should come from your shoulders and back. Keep your wrists straight during the move. At the top of the lift, your elbows should point back—or as close to that direction as you can manage.
- **Pause for a breath.**
- **1-2-3-Down:** Slowly lower the dumbbells to the starting position.
- **Pause for a breath, then repeat.**

Where you will feel the effort

In your upper back, upper arms, and shoulders, as well as your lower back and abdomen; in your thighs, because these muscles work to hold your body stable while you do the exercise.

Sets and reps

Do eight repetitions for one set. Rest for a minute or two and do a second set.

Notes

Caution: if you have osteoporosis, talk with your doctor before you do this exercise.

In the beginning, your elbows may point to the sides. As you become slimmer, stronger, and more flexible, you'll be able to point your elbows farther back. Similarly, if your abdomen is large, you might have trouble leaning forward. Just bend as far as is comfortable and perform the lift.

- Make sure your head, neck, and back are in a straight line. Don't flex or arch your back.
- Though you're supposed to bring your shoulder blades together, don't scrunch your shoulders up toward your ears.
- Move slowly.
- Don't hold your breath.
- Check for tension, and relax.

Calf Raise

Toned calf muscles give curves as well as strength to your lower legs. This exercise also strengthens your ankle joints and makes them more flexible. These changes improve your balance and add power to every move you make on your feet, whether it's walking, climbing stairs, or cross-country skiing.

As your calves get stronger and your balance improves, try to perform this exercise with less assistance from your hands. Eventually, you may be able to do it with hands poised above the chair but not holding on.

Starting position

Stand behind a sturdy chair that has a back high enough for you to hold for balance. Stand with feet shoulder-width apart, fingertips resting lightly on the back of the chair.

The move

- **1-2-3-Up:** Slowly raise yourself up as high as you can on the balls of your feet.
- **Hold for three seconds.**
- **1-2-3-Down:** Slowly lower your heels back to the starting position.
- **Pause for a breath, then repeat.**

Where you will feel the effort

In your ankles, feet, and calves.

Sets and reps

Do eight repetitions for one set. Rest for a minute or two and do a second set.

Notes

◆ Check your posture; make sure
  you stand up straight.

◆ Move slowly.

◆ Don't hold your breath.

◆ Check for tension, and relax—
  make sure your knee joints are
  relaxed, not locked or
  hyperextended.

Seated Fly

Strong, shapely shoulders look beautiful in a bathing suit or tank top. This exercise really concentrates on the shoulder muscles. Stronger shoulder muscles contribute to good posture, and they help with heavy lifting. The move can be a little tricky to coordinate at first, but it's easy once you learn it.

Starting position

Sit forward in the chair with your feet flat on the floor shoulder-width (40 to 45 centimetres/15 to 18 inches) apart. With your upper arms against your sides, grasp one dumbbell in each hand, palms facing your thighs. Bend your elbows slightly. Your hands will be just in front of your hips, on the outside of your thighs.

▼ ▼ ▼ ▼ ▼ ▼ ▼ ▼ ▼ ▼ ▼ ▼ ▼ ▼ ▼ ▼ ▼ ▼

The move

- **1-2-3-Up:** Slowly lift your upper arms straight out to the sides, maintaining the same slight bend in your elbow. At the end of the lift, your upper arms will be parallel to the floor and straight out to the sides of your shoulders. Your forearms—still slightly bent—will also be parallel to the floor.
- **Pause for a breath.**
- **1-2-3-Down:** In a smooth motion, lower your arms back to the starting position.
- **Pause for a breath, then repeat.**

Where you will feel the effort

In your shoulders and upper arms.

Sets and reps

Do eight repetitions for one set. Rest for a minute or two and do a second set.

Notes

This exercise can be confusing at first, but the move is very fluid and easy once you learn it. Most women need to use a lighter dumbbell for this exercise than for the others, because this muscle is usually weaker.

- Throughout the move, keep your elbow just slightly bent. The effort should come from your shoulder muscles.
- Don't scrunch your shoulders.
- Don't let your arms come above shoulder height.
- Move slowly.
- Don't hold your breath.
- Check for tension, and relax.

ARM CURL

Women love this exercise—which strengthens the biceps—because it
gets fast results. You'll feel the difference when you're lifting shopping
bags or acing a tennis serve. And your arms will look great too.

▼ ▼ ▼ ▼ ▼ ▼ ▼ ▼ ▼ ▼ ▼ ▼ ▼ ▼ ▼ ▼ ▼

Starting position

Stand with your feet shoulder-width apart, with your arms down at your sides holding the dumbbells. Palms should face in, towards your legs.

The move

♦ **1-2-3-Up:** Keeping your elbows gently pressed against your sides, raise the dumbbells by bringing your forearms up. The dumbbells should move from your sides to the front of your shoulders in one smooth motion. Your elbows will bend; your forearms will rotate; and your wrists will remain straight. At the end of the move, the dumbbells will be at shoulder height, parallel to the floor, with your palms facing your shoulders.

♦ **Pause for a breath.**

♦ **1-2-3-Down:** Lower your arms, smoothly rotating your forearms so the dumbbells return to the starting position, with palms facing in. Keep your elbows gently anchored at your sides through the entire movement.

♦ **Pause for a breath, then repeat.**

Where you will feel the effort

In your upper arms.

Sets and reps

Do eight repetitions for one set. Rest for a minute or two and do a second set.

Notes

♦ Maintain good posture; don't arch your back.

♦ Don't bend your wrists.

♦ Keep your elbows anchored at your sides.

♦ Move slowly.

♦ Don't hold your breath.

♦ Check for tension, and relax.

STRETCH

A brief stretch after a strength-training session helps prevent injury and contributes to flexibility. If you're doing aerobic exercise and strength training in the same workout, begin with aerobics to warm your muscles, then strength train—and save the stretching for the end. It's a wonderful way to relax after vigorous exercise.

The basic instructions for stretching are very simple. Get into the position, extending your muscles as far as you comfortably can. Hold the stretch for 20 to 30 seconds, breathing normally. During the stretch, gently try to extend the position, but never go to the point of discomfort. Try to relax your muscles as much as possible—the more you relax, the more your muscles will be able to stretch.

Shoulder Stretch

This move stretches the muscles of your shoulders and upper arms. Stand with your feet shoulder-width apart, arms at your sides. Extend your arms straight behind your body, pulling them back and up as high as you can. You may clasp your hands together, if you're able to do so.

Quadriceps Stretch

Stand next to the chair. Holding on with your left hand, bend your right knee so your right leg comes up behind you. Grasp your ankle and hold it, pointing your knee down (or as close to down as possible). Hold the stretch for 20 to 30 seconds, then release. Repeat, switching so that you hold on to the chair with your right hand and bend your left knee.

Note: at first, you may not be able to reach your ankle when you bend your knee and raise your leg behind you. In that case, just bend your knee and bring your lower leg back; keep your thigh perpendicular to the ground and your lower leg parallel to the floor.

Lower Back and Hamstring Stretch

Sit forward in a chair with your feet flat on the floor. Your thigh should form a right angle with your lower leg. Slide your right leg forward, keeping your heel on the floor, until your right knee is straight, but not locked. Your ankle should be relaxed. Extend both arms, pointing your fingers toward your right foot. Bend as far towards your right foot as you comfortably can. Hold the stretch for 20 seconds, then release. Repeat, this time extending your left leg.

▼ ▼ ▼ ▼ ▼ ▼ ▼ ▼ ▼ ▼ ▼ ▼ ▼ ▼ ▼ ▼ ▼

Lower Leg and Ankle Stretch

Sit in a chair with your feet flat on the floor. Extend your legs slightly so that your heels are 2 to 5 centimetres (1 to 2 inches) off the floor. Flex your toes up and bend your ankles back towards you as much as you can. Hold the stretch for 20 to 30 seconds, then point your toes down and bend your feet away from you as far as possible. Hold the stretch for 20 to 30 seconds.

CREATING AN INDIVIDUALISED PROGRAMME

You've learned the moves. The next step is to turn the exercises into an *individualised programme* that will increase your strength. This programme will be simple—but not easy! To become strong, you must train at a challenging level. As you become stronger, you'll need to adjust to maintain that challenge. Using the right weights or version for each exercise is the key to both safety and success. If you overdo it, you'll find the programme unnecessarily difficult. On the other hand, if you expect too little of yourself, you won't see the kind of progress that makes strength training so exciting.

WHERE TO START

The heaviest weight you can lift just once is your maximum strength capacity. You'll be working out at 70 to 80 per cent of your maximum. This means the lifts are well within your ability, yet the effort is great enough to improve your strength. For safety's sake, you'll start at a level that's considerably lower—no more than 50 to 60 per cent—while you're learning the moves.

- If you're already following the *Strong Women Stay Young* programme or another strength-training programme, but you want to switch to the exercises in this book, start with weights that are the same as or lower than what you're using now. For a familiar exercise, use your customary weight; if the exercise is new, use your lightest weight and increase after a session or two.

- If you've never strength trained before (or haven't done so recently) and are in good health, start with 1.35-kilogram (3-lb) weights.

- If you have health concerns, discuss the programme with your doctor before you start. One option to consider is beginning the exercises without weights.

Your first few sessions probably will seem a little too easy, but in my experience that's helpful when you're mastering proper form. Within a few weeks, you'll reach the right intensity. After that, you'll add weight or move to the next version as your muscles strengthen. The programme will always be right for your body.

How to Evaluate Your Effort

The scale—inspired by the Borg Exercise Intensity Scale that many researchers use—will help you recognise when you're working out at the right intensity.

The right effort for strength training is Level 4. You should find the weight moderately difficult to lift the first time, but well within your capability. By the third or fourth lift, it should seem heavier. Ideally you should be able to perform the eighth lift in good form, but feel that if you didn't stop and rest your muscles, you couldn't continue.

Working out at Level 3 (except for the first few weeks) is not sufficiently challenging; it will increase your endurance, but not your strength. On the other hand, training at Level 5 is risky—if the effort is too great, you won't be able to maintain proper form and you might injure yourself.

With the exercises that use body weight, you won't be able to adjust your effort quite so precisely. Aim to move to the next higher version as soon as you can do so without exceeding Level 4 intensity. If you are unsure, wait. It's better to progress more slowly than to work your muscles too hard.

Finding the Right Challenge

I've given you a very conservative starting point—just 1 kilogram in most cases—so you can focus on your form, on breathing and relaxing, and on establishing the slow rhythm of lifting and lowering a weight. By the fourth week you should be training at Level 4 intensity.

Week 1:

Stay at the starting level for all three sessions to learn the exercises, even if it's too easy. If your first session seems too hard, or if your muscles are very uncomfortable afterward, do the exercises without weights.

Week 2:

For the exercises that use dumbbells, add the weight per session or per few sessions, as needed, to increase effort to Level 4. However, if your muscles

EXERCISE INTENSITY SCALE FOR STRENGTH TRAINING	
LEVEL	**DESCRIPTION OF EFFORT**
1	Very easy: too easy to be noticed; like lifting a pencil.
2	Easy: can be felt, but isn't fatiguing; like carrying a book.
3	Moderate: fatiguing only if prolonged; like carrying a full handbag that seems heavier as the day goes on.
4	Hard: more than moderate at first, and becoming difficult by the time you complete six or seven repetitions. You can make the effort eight times in good form, but need to rest afterwards.
5	Extremely hard: requires all your strength, like lifting a piece of heavy furniture that you can only lift once, if at all.

are sore, continue with the same weight or, if the discomfort is bothersome, decrease the weight. You may find that you need to add weights on some exercises but not others. That's normal, because the strengths of different muscles vary.

Week 3:

Aim to be working out at Level 4 on all the exercises by the end of this week. (You'll also begin your aerobics programme this week—more about that in Chapter 8.) Don't be surprised if you're using different dumbbells for different exercises.

WORKING TOWARDS GOALS

After the initial adjustment, try to increase the weight for each exercise every week. Of course, you shouldn't attempt to work out at Level 5. But you'll make more progress if you push yourself to stay at the top of the Level 4 range rather than waiting so long to increase the weight that your effort has dropped to Level 3.

Sometimes you'll find yourself between dumbbells or versions—what you're doing seems too easy, but the next step up is too difficult. The best way to make the transition is to use your current weight or version for the first set, then move up for the second set. After a few sessions, you'll be ready to do both sets in good form at the more challenging intensity.

Weekly changes won't always be possible. Also, you'll soon see that progress is easier with some exercises than with others. The wide range of individual responses always fascinates me. Some women move forward

STRENGTH-TRAINING GOALS

EXERCISE	20 TO 49 YEARS OLD	50 TO 69 YEARS OLD	70 YEARS AND OLDER
Chair stand	Version 2	Version 2	Version 2
Overhead press	5–7.5 kilos (12–16½ lb)	4–5 kilos (9–11 lb)	3–4 kilos (6½–9 lb)
Bent-over row	5–7.5 kilos (12–16½ lb)	4–5 kilos (9–11 lb)	3–4 kilos (6½–9 lb)
Calf raise	No hands	No hands	No hands
Seated fly	3–4 kilos (6½–9 lb)	2–3 kilos (4½–6½ lb)	1–3 kilos (2–6½ lb)
Arm curl	5–7.5 kilos (12–16½ lb)	4–5 kilos (9–11 lb)	3–4 kilos (6½–9 lb)

rapidly; others advance more slowly. There are certain common patterns, though. Most people find the arm curl considerably easier than the seated fly and overhead press. That's because the arm curl uses the biceps muscles, which tend to be a lot stronger than the triceps in the back of the arm (used for the overhead press) and the shoulder muscles (used for the seated fly). Don't be discouraged—all of your muscle groups will become stronger.

The table on page 141 shows strength goals by age and exercise. When you're training at these levels, you will have obtained most of the health benefits you can expect from a strengthening programme—provided you keep it up. Most women reach these goals after six to nine months on this programme, or at least come close.

These goals are by no means upper limits. Studies that follow people for as long as two years find that they keep improving, though of course the changes become very slow. How much further you go is up to you. My personal preference is to maintain healthy levels, rather than struggling to surpass them.

WHEN YOU'RE READY FOR MORE

I've included two optional extra exercises to further strengthen the muscles of your back and abdomen, as well as your lower body. All use your own weight for resistance. I encourage you to include them in your programme, but not right away. You'll have a lot to learn when you start the *Strong Women Stay Slim* programme—the basic strengthening exercises, plus your aerobics exercises and the food plan. That's plenty for the first four weeks. After that, you can begin adding the extra moves if you wish. Perform the new moves right after the chair stands, then continue with the other five exercises of the basic six, and end with your stretches.

Pelvic Tilt

This exercise is a classic—and for good reason. One simple move firms and strengthens your entire midsection: buttocks, thighs, abdomen, and back. It's a perfect complement to the basic programme. You can do the exercise on a firm mattress or padded bench if you'd rather not get down on the floor.

Starting position

Lie on your back with your knees bent and feet flat on the floor, shoulder-width apart. Your arms should be at your sides and relaxed, with palms flat.

The move

- **1-2-3-Up:** Slowly roll your pelvis off the floor—first your hips, then your waist, and finally your lower back. Your midsection should form a straight line from your knees to your upper back. Your shoulders will remain on the floor.
- **Pause for a breath.**

- **1-2-3-Down:** Slowly roll back to the starting position, lowering first your back, then your waist, and finally your hips.

- **Pause for a breath, then repeat.**

Where you will feel the effort

In the front and back of your thighs, buttocks, abdomen, and lower back.

Sets and reps

Do eight repetitions for one set. Rest briefly and do another set of eight repetitions.

Notes

Caution: this exercise puts pressure on your upper back. If you have osteoporosis or back problems, check with your doctor before trying it.

- If you find the move uncomfortable, don't roll quite so far back.

- When you lower yourself, your movement should be controlled; don't drop onto the floor.

- Move smoothly and slowly.

- Don't hold your breath.

- Check for tension, and relax—make sure your toes are relaxed.

FRONT LEG RAISE

Here's an excellent thigh-shaper. The bonus is added leg strength, which helps when you're walking, playing sports, or rising from a chair.

Starting position

Sit on the floor and lean back slightly. Put your hands on the floor behind your

buttocks to help support your upper body. Extend your legs straight in front of you. Put a rolled-up towel under your right knee to keep you from locking your knee. Your left knee should be bent, with your left foot on the floor next to your right leg, just above the ankle.

The move

- **1-2-3-Up:** Slowly lift your right leg as high as possible—this may be as little as 10 centimetres (4 inches) in the beginning, up to 40 centimetres (15 inches) when you become stronger and more flexible. Keep your right leg straight, with the foot relaxed and toes pointing up.
- **Pause for a breath.**
- **1-2-3-Down:** Slowly lower your right leg to the floor.
- **Pause for a breath, then repeat.**

Where you will feel the effort

In the front and back of the raised thigh, and in your lower back.

Sets and reps

Repeat until you have done eight lifts with your right leg; then do eight lifts with your left leg. That's one set. Rest for a minute or two, then do a second set.

Notes

As you become stronger, try to lift your leg higher off the floor.

- The movement should be slow and controlled; don't let your leg drop.
- Don't round your back or slump your shoulders.
- Don't hold your breath.
- Check for tension, and relax—make sure your toes are relaxed.

TO READERS OF
STRONG WOMEN STAY YOUNG

If you've been following the programme in my first book, you may be puzzled to see that the exercises in this book are different, and that I recommend three strength-training sessions per week instead of two. And perhaps you're wondering whether you should continue with your *SWSY* routine or make a switch. So I want to explain the differences and make a few suggestions.

The *Strong Women Stay Slim* programme calls for three strength-training sessions per week because it's designed for weight loss—an extra session revs up your metabolism even more and helps preserve muscle and bone as you lose weight. Because you're doing three sessions and also aerobic exercise, I streamlined the strength training. That's why I didn't include exercises with ankle weights.

If you've been following the programme in *SWSY* and want to continue, by all means do so. But if you're losing weight, consider doing three *SWSY* sessions per week instead of two.

If you'd like to combine the two programmes, here are some guidelines so you don't overwork the same muscles:

◆ **Arm exercises:** Do the biceps curls following either *SWSY* or this book. Do either the overhead triceps from *SWSY* or the overhead press from this book. And do all the other arm exercises—the bentover row and seated fly from this book, and the upward row from *SWSY*. If you want to omit one of these three, drop the upward row.

◆ **Leg exercises:** If you want to continue working out with ankle weights, stick with the leg exercises in *SWSY*. You can add the chair stands from this book if you wish—indeed, I suggested using them for a warm-up in *SWSY*. If you prefer not to use the ankle weights, just do the chair stands and the calf raises from this book; add the heel stands from *SWSY* if you wish.

EASE YOURSELF
INTO FITNESS

When I'm under stress and my shoulders are up around my ears, I go for a swim or a run. It gets all the tension out. My energy level is much higher; I feel much better; my back doesn't hurt. I'm fitting into things again. I had been size 16 going on 18. Now I'm almost in size 14.

—Nancy

◆ ◆ ◆

A erobic activity is one of the great health tonics—and a terrific calorie burner. Once your body is strong and fit, it's a joy to be physically active.

I realise that you may be unaccustomed to aerobic exercise. If so, you can start slowly. You don't have to begin the aerobic portion of the *Strong Women Stay Slim* programme until the third week, and your first session can be as brief as 10 minutes. From this modest beginning, you'll steadily progress until, by the tenth week, you will have reached the standard for vigorous physical activity suggested by the American College of Sports Medicine, the US Surgeon General, and the US Centers for Disease Control and Prevention. This is no small feat: according to recent surveys, at least three-quarters of women in the western world don't meet the recommended minimum. In addition, I expect you'll feel more energetic and be more active throughout the day, which is important for weight loss too.

AEROBIC OPTIONS

I think it's helpful to have one "daily bread" exercise—something you can count on doing three to six times a week, which easily becomes a routine part of your life. Any sustained activity that elevates your heart rate is acceptable for this programme.

If you're already doing exercise of this kind, that's great! Just continue, adjusting as necessary to progress toward the fitness goals described later in the chapter. If you've been sedentary, I suggest you select one aerobic activity for the first few weeks. Once you become familiar with it, you can expand your repertoire. Variety will prevent boredom; also, different activities strengthen different muscles.

Women often ask me, "What's the best aerobic activity?" My answer: **The best activity is one that you enjoy and is easy for you to do regularly**.

My mother, who's 70 years old and lives in Vermont, cross-country skis five days a week during the winter and mountain bikes in the summer. Cross-country skiing is my favourite way to exercise but, unlike my mum, I can't do it frequently. Because I've been a competitive athlete I need a strenuous activity to maintain my fitness level, so my "daily bread" exercise is running. I run (or do something equally demanding) three to five times a week. In addition, I'm physically active every day—climbing stairs, walking, playing with my kids.

For many women, brisk walking is the ideal aerobic activity because it fits so easily into their lives. But if you don't enjoy walking, or find it painful or impractical, it's not the best exercise for you. Fortunately, there are many other options.

♦ ♦ ♦

I live in a hot climate with a long summer, and a swim before dinner revives me. I swim various strokes to make sure I'm training all my muscles. It's a wonderful spirit-lifter. Sometimes I think out

a problem while I'm doing laps. Other times I don't think at all. Even though it's hard work, when I'm finished I always feel relaxed, as if the worries of the day have dissolved in the water.
　　—Barbara

◆　◆　◆

I have a painful heel spur in my left foot, and I can't do weight bearing exercise for more than 15 minutes at a time. But I can cycle.
　　—Jane

◆　◆　◆

I use cardiovascular machines—mainly a treadmill and a recumbent stair climber—at a health club. I like the detailed feedback I get from machines, because I can see even tiny progress, and that's very encouraging. Also, I like working out at a gym: it's air-conditioned, it's safe, and there's a bathroom nearby.
　　—Sarah

◆　◆　◆

GENERAL INSTRUCTIONS

A few basic measures will make your aerobic workouts more effective, safer, and much more enjoyable.

DRESS FOR SUCCESS

Comfortable clothes keep your workout pleasurable, and even protect you. Some women get a boost from stylish exercise gear, but if you prefer to keep it simple, a loose cotton T-shirt and shorts or leggings are just fine.

- ◆ Dress for the weather. On cold days, wear layers that you can peel off as your body warms up. When it's warm, wear light colours outdoors (dark colours absorb heat from the sun). Select cotton garments or look for new materials that help draw sweat away from your skin.

♦ Dress for safety. If you're working out on equipment, wear clothing that can't get caught in moving parts. Use all recommended safety gear—a helmet if you're cycling, or reflecting strips on clothing if you walk at night.

♦ Protect yourself from the sun if you exercise outdoors. Wear sunscreen and sunglasses, plus a hat with a visor.

♦ Wear a supportive, comfortable bra that allows free movement.

♦ Wear clean socks made from an absorbent material. Make sure they fit well, with no folds or seams that chafe your feet. Keep your toenails clipped so they don't push up against another toe or the end of your shoe.

♦ Select shoes that fit well and that are appropriate for your activity. Good athletic shoes can be expensive, but they're worth it because they help prevent injuries and discomfort. Note: if your shoes are a year old, chances are they need replacement or repair. Examine footwear at least once a month. When you become active, you'll find that shoes wear out more quickly.

SELECT SAFE SURROUNDINGS

If you exercise outdoors, take sensible precautions. Avoid unsafe neighbourhoods and dangerous traffic. If the weather is wet, watch for slippery surfaces when you're cycling or running. Try to find an exercise companion—or at least stick to well-populated routes—especially at night.

CHECK THE EQUIPMENT

If you're using equipment—bicycle, stationary cycle, treadmill, etc.— give it a quick look-over before each workout to make sure it's in good repair. Follow all maintenance suggestions in the manual.

CAUTION

Remember to take the PAR-Q (see page 98) before you begin this or any other exercise programme.

If you follow the instructions in this book, it's extremely unlikely that you'll ever experience any of the symptoms below. But if you do, use common sense: stop training immediately. And if the symptom persists, contact your medical caregiver.

♦ Chest pain or pressure

♦ Dizziness or light-headedness

♦ Nausea

♦ Sweating not explained by physical effort or by hot flushes

♦ Any unusual or worsening pain—for instance, pain in a joint; or pain in the jaw or in the arm or shoulder that's not caused by muscle fatigue

DRINK PLENTY OF WATER

During aerobic activity, your body requires extra water. You're evaporating water—in the form of perspiration—to keep cool. You're also releasing additional moisture through respiration, because you're breathing more rapidly. And your stepped-up metabolism is creating waste products that need to be flushed away. Consequently, for top performance during aerobic exercise, your body needs to be well hydrated.

To ensure that you're getting enough, drink at least one glass of water during the hour before your workout. Then drink another glass or two within the 45 minutes following aerobic activity. If an activity is prolonged—for instance, if you're taking a long hike or spending an afternoon gardening—drink a cup of water every hour or so. Your need for water will be even greater on hot days, when your body has to work harder to stay cool.

A simple way to monitor hydration is by glancing at your urine when you go to the toilet. Ideally, urine should be very pale yellow, almost clear. If it's dark, you're probably dehydrated.

LIMIT DISTRACTIONS

Exercise can be more enjoyable if you're listening to music or conversing with a friend. Some women like to read or watch TV while they ride their stationary cycle. That's fine, so long as the distraction doesn't interfere with a safe and effective workout. However, I don't recommend it at the beginning, when you're learning to use the equipment.

Two cautions if you wear headphones to listen to a personal stereo radio/player: keep the volume low enough to be kind to your ears; and if you're outdoors, make sure you can hear what's happening around you.

WARM UP

Muscles work best when they're warm: they're more elastic and have a better supply of blood. So it's important to warm your muscles before you place heavy demands on them. This is especially true for older people and those with cardiovascular disease.

A warm-up need not be elaborate. Just begin your exercise at a slow, easy pace, rather than at full speed. Take five minutes to reach your target intensity. This gradual transition from a resting to an active state gives your body time to adjust.

COOL DOWN AND STRETCH

After aerobic exercise, it's tempting to fall into a chair or to tear off your sweaty clothes and stand under the shower. Not yet! Your body needs to cool down first, and your muscles need a stretch.

When you're exercising at the proper intensity, your heart is pumping, your blood vessels are dilated, and your muscles are contracting to push blood back from your extremities to your heart. If you stop too abruptly, your heart is still pumping blood out, but your muscles are not returning it. This could make you feel dizzy or faint; in rare cases it could even cause serious heart irregularities. The problem can be exacerbated by heat, which is why a gradual cool-down is especially important if you plan to visit the sauna or steam room after exercising.

The cool-down is just as simple as the warm-up, only in reverse: over a five-minute period, slow your pace to the equivalent of a slow walk. Afterwards you can do your strengthening exercises if you're combining the two into a single workout session.

End your exercise session with a stretch. Stretching is particularly important after an aerobic workout because most aerobic activities work your muscles at high intensity, but through only a limited range of motion. If you don't stretch afterwards, you can actually decrease your flexibility. The four simple stretches described on pages 134–137 in Chapter 7 prevent that problem—and they feel great!

HOW TO GAUGE AEROBIC EFFORT

The key to getting results from aerobic exercise, just as with strength training, is to work out at the right intensity. When you do strength training, you use a weight you can lift eight times in good form—but no more—before you have to rest. You'll be aiming for a similar kind of challenge when you do aerobic exercise, but you'll use different indicators, including your heart rate.

When you do aerobic exercise in this programme, your heart will work at about 60 to 70 per cent of its maximum most of the time. This is safely within your capability but high enough to give your cardiovascular system a good workout. How do you know you're at the right level? In the laboratory, we use heart-rate monitoring and a 20-point exercise-intensity scale to measure aerobic effort. But in most cases, you can get all the information you need by referring to a very simple intensity scale or by checking your pulse.

ESTIMATING EXERCISE INTENSITY

The easiest way to measure aerobic effort is with a subjective scale that describes how you're feeling as you exercise. You can use the scale at any point in your workout, and you don't need special apparatus. Though this system generally works well, I encourage you also to take your pulse a few times (I'll tell you how in a minute), to make sure your impressions match your actual heart rate.

The *Strong Women Stay Slim* aerobics programme calls for Level 3 effort. But I hope you'll also do considerably more Level 2 activity as you

Exercise Intensity Scale for Aerobic Activity

Level	Description of effort
1—Sedentary	No perceived effort; standing, sitting, or lying down.
2—Active This level contributes to overall health and burns more calories than being sedentary.	Easy, sustainable movement that causes a small increase in heart and breathing rate and doesn't raise a sweat (unless the weather is hot); strolling, gardening, slow dancing, golfing.
3—Aerobic training You should exercise at this level to condition your heart and lungs.	Somewhat hard movement that elevates the heart rate to 60 to 70 per cent of maximum most of the time, ranging up to 80 per cent. Breathing is more rapid, though it's possible to converse with only slightly altered speech; perspiration appears after about five to fifteen minutes, depending on air temperature.
4—Athletic training This is a more advanced level of aerobic conditioning that might become an appropriate goal after the ten-week programme.	Hard effort that elevates the heart rate to 70 to 80 per cent most of the time, ranging up to 90 per cent of maximum. Breathing is rapid but not laboured—it's possible to converse, though faster breathing causes interruptions; perspiration starts within five to ten minutes, depending on air temperature; fatigue increases as the workout continues and you will feel a need to stop by the end.
5—Over-exertion Not recommended!	Excessive effort: heart pounds to the point of discomfort or nausea; breathing is too rapid to permit speech.

become stronger and more fit. The more active you are, the more calories and fat you burn. Indeed, **if you simply add half an hour of Level 2 activity a day for a year, without making any changes in your diet, you'll lose about 4.5 kilograms (10 lb).**

Once you're familiar with the intensity scale, it will help you stay in touch with your body during your workouts. That's very important, because you'll need to adjust your exercise sessions over time. As you become fitter, you'll increase your pace to maintain the right level of challenge. If you catch a cold or miss sleep and feel temporarily run down, you'll need to slow down for a day or more. These adjustments are easy and natural if you've learned how to listen to your body.

MEASURING YOUR HEART RATE

Heart-rate monitors can be purchased at sporting goods stores, but the good monitors cost between £60 and £300. Monitors are built into some gym equipment. Many women find them fun to use and like the precise, detailed feedback they provide. But you can get the same information without spending any money by taking your radial (wrist) pulse. (Note: don't take your pulse at your neck, by pressing on your carotid artery—that could impede blood flow to your brain.)

To take your radial pulse, all you need is a clock or watch with a second hand.

♦ Position yourself so you can see your watch or the clock.

♦ Bend your right arm at the elbow and hold your right hand out.

- Holding the forefinger and middle finger of your left hand together, touch them to the base of your right thumb.

- Very slowly, slide the fingers across your wrist, moving them parallel to the top of your right arm. Your left fingers will cross the bones of your right wrist, then you'll feel a narrow hollow in your right forearm between the bone on top and the tendons below.

- Press firmly when you're at the hollow. You should be able to feel your radial pulse. It may help to bend your right wrist back slightly.

- Watching the clock, count the number of beats you feel for fifteen seconds. Multiply the number by four to get your heart rate—in beats per minute.

During an exercise session, you'll have to slow down a little to check your pulse. This will decrease your heart rate, so practise a few times to get the knack of taking the measurement quickly. There are two good times to check your heart rate: when you're five minutes into your aerobic activity, and at the end before you cool down. And you can check it whenever you want to know how hard you're working.

TARGET HEART RATE FOR AEROBIC EXERCISE

Your **target heart rate** is 60 to 80 per cent of your maximum heart rate. During aerobic exercise sessions you'll work out at 60 to 70 per cent most of the time, occasionally going up to 75 or 80 per cent. Use this formula to estimate your maximum heart rate (or use the chart on the next page):

MAXIMUM HEART RATE = 220 minus your age in years
TARGET HEART RATE = 60 per cent to 80 per cent of maximum heart rate

Example:

> Lois is 40. Her maximum heart rate is 180, which is 220 minus 40.
>
> 60 per cent of 180 (.6 × 180) is 108 beats per minute.
>
> 70 per cent of 180 (.7 × 180) is 126 beats per minute.
>
> 80 per cent of 180 (.8 × 180) is 144 beats per minute.

When Lois exercises, she'll maintain a heart rate of 108 to 144 beats per minute, staying between 108 and 126 most of the time.

TARGET HEART RATE
(BEATS PER MINUTE)

MAINTAIN A HEART RATE BETWEEN 60% AND 80% OF MAXIMUM, STAYING BETWEEN 60% AND 70% MOST OF THE TIME.

Age	60%	70%	80%	90%
20	120	140	160	180
25	117	137	156	176
30	114	133	152	171
35	111	130	148	167
40	108	126	144	162
45	105	123	140	158
50	102	119	136	153
55	99	116	132	149
60	96	112	128	144
65	93	109	124	140
70	90	105	120	135
75	87	102	116	131
80	84	98	112	126

WHAT ELSE AFFECTS YOUR HEART RATE?

Your heart responds to changes in your activity. As you work harder, it beats faster; when you slow down, your heart slows down too. During outdoor exercise, your heart rate will vary as you go up and down hills or stop at a traffic light. But your heart rate can be affected by other factors as well:

- If you're using a pacemaker or taking drugs to keep your heart rate steady.

- If you're taking medications that can raise or lower your heart rate, such as cold remedies, appetite suppressants, or calcium channel blockers for blood pressure.

- If you've recently consumed caffeine, which can raise your heart rate. Caffeine is found not only in coffee and tea, but also in some soft drinks and in medications taken for headach and other pain.

In these situations, use the exercise intensity scale to assess your effort rather than relying on your pulse. When in doubt, always err on the side of caution and slow your pace. Also, if you have concerns, talk to your doctor.

TEN WEEKS TO AEROBIC FITNESS

As you know by now, I'm a strong believer in the power of slow starts and gradual but steady improvement. Nevertheless, you may be surprised by how little is expected of you at first on the *Strong Women Stay Slim* programme: no aerobic exercise for the first two weeks, and just 10 minutes the week after that. While this is a slower beginning than some physiologists might advise, there are good reasons to wait.

First, if you've been sedentary, your muscles, tendons, and ligaments may be weak. Two weeks of strength training will make them stronger, so your first aerobic workouts will be easier and safer. Second, there's a lot going on when you start this programme: you're learning the strengthening exercises, beginning to keep food records, and changing your diet. I don't want you to ever feel overwhelmed. If you begin gradually and progress steadily, you can painlessly ease yourself into a healthy lifestyle. When you look back ten weeks from now, you'll be astonished and delighted by how far you've come.

How Fit Are You Now? Take the Walking Test

If you can comfortably walk a kilometre (½ mile), I encourage you to take the simple walking test below to estimate your aerobic fitness before you begin the programme. You'll walk a kilometre as fast as you can. Over the coming weeks and months, you'll be able to repeat the test and track your fitness progress. I developed this test from my experience working with women of different ages and abilities, and by reviewing current medical research on walking and fitness levels.

Step 1: Take the PAR-Q questionnaire on page 98 to learn whether you need to check with your doctor first. If you're very out of shape, or if your mobility is limited by arthritis or another condition, skip the test for now. You may be able to take it in a few weeks, after you've gradually increased your strength and cardiovascular fitness.

Step 2: Find a track or a road with a measured kilometre where walking is safe. If you prefer a track, call your local high school, college, or community centre to ask about using their facility; find out how many laps equal a kilometre.

Step 3: Select a day when the weather is good. Dress as you would for a workout, in comfortable clothes and sturdy shoes. Bring along a stopwatch plus a pencil and paper.

Step 4: Before the test, warm up for five minutes by walking at a moderate pace.

Step 5: Begin the test. Note the time and walk one kilometre as fast as you comfortably can. If you regularly run or jog, you may do so for all or part of the test.

Step 6: Record your time as you finish the kilometre.

Step 7: Cool down by walking slowly for five minutes.

Step 8: Check the chart to determine your fitness level.

Don't be discouraged if you fall into a low category or can't even complete the test. That's not surprising if you haven't been exercising, especially if you're overweight. If you start working out regularly, you *will* improve—and that will be a great accomplishment. Indeed, just completing the test can be a major achievement for a woman who was extremely sedentary before she started the programme.

HOW TO FIND THE RIGHT PROGRESS TRACK

Depending on your present fitness, you'll follow one of three different progress tracks. Use the test results, or if you didn't take the test, approximate your level of fitness with the following table:

WHAT'S YOUR PROGRESS TRACK?

PROGRESS TRACK	FITNESS TEST SCORE	FITNESS APPROXIMATION
Fast	Excellent	"I can briskly walk, jog or run a km."
Medium	Good	"I can walk a km without resting, but couldn't run or jog."
Slow	Poor or unable to take the test	"I couldn't walk a km without resting."

Aerobic Fitness
Minutes to walk or run a kilometre ($^1/_2$ mile)

Age	Excellent	Good	Poor
20–39	less than 7:30	7:30–8:59	11 or more
40–49	less than 8	9:00–10:29	11:45 or more
50–59	less than 8:30	10:30–11:59	13 or more
60–69	less than 9	11:00–12:29	13:45 or more
70 and older	less than 9:30	12:30–13:59	14 or more

If you're not sure where you belong on this scale, select the lower category. While going too fast could cause problems, progressing a little less rapidly than you might have is no cause for concern. At the end of ten weeks, you'll be at the same point no matter how quickly you got there.

Remember: if you're already doing aerobic exercise, you don't have to stop. Keep working out at your present level, but pay attention to the intensity level and to the time you spend. At first, you may be far ahead of the weekly progress goals I suggest below, but as time passes, you'll probably find that the goals in the table catch up. From that point on, continue with the *Strong Women Stay Slim* programme.

WEEKLY GOALS FOR AEROBIC ACTIVITY

Unless you're already exercising, you don't have to begin aerobic activity component of the *Strong Women Stay Slim* programme until the third week. At that point, you'll do a 10-minute workout at Level 3 intensity, plus warm-up, cool-down, and stretch. Thereafter you'll gradually extend the aerobic sessions to 30 minutes.

If you're already fit, you'll progress more rapidly. Use the chart that follows to set your goals, and be sure to keep logs (see pages 215–216) to track your improvement.

Do at least three Level 3 aerobic workouts per week—but no more than six. Your body needs a day of rest. Studies find that people who overdo aerobic exercise by training seven days a week have more injuries than those who take a weekly break.

If you want to do strength training and aerobic activity during the same workout, it's best to do the aerobic exercise first so that your muscles are warmed up. Follow this sequence:

- ◆ Warm-up
- ◆ Aerobic activity
- ◆ Cool-down
- ◆ Strength training
- ◆ Stretches (from Chapter 7, pages 134–137).

I'm frequently asked whether it's okay to break a 20-minute session into two 10-minute sessions a day. Yes, it is. In fact, the newest research shows that splitting your sessions into 10-minute segments is just as effective for improving cardiovascular fitness. Because you still need to warm up and cool

Use the chart on page 161 to determine your progress track.

WEEKLY PROGRESS GOALS
MINUTES OF LEVEL 3 AEROBIC ACTIVITY,
THREE TO SIX DAYS PER WEEK

WEEK	SLOW TRACK	MEDIUM TRACK	FAST TRACK
1	0	0	0
2	0	0	0
3	10	10	10
4	10	10	15
5	10	15	20
6	15	15	20
7	15	20	25
8	20	25	30
9	25	30	30
10	30	30	30

down for each mini-session, you actually end up exercising more throughout the day.

Which way is best—one long session or several short ones? Your preference should be the deciding factor. Dianne enjoys short walks tucked into her busy day. When she has an appointment near a nice place to walk, she arrives 15 minutes early so she can take a brisk walk. She builds walking time into everyday errands, such as going to the post office. But Jayne says, "I like to get into my exercise clothes, work out, shower, and change—and be done with it."

Women also ask if they can move ahead more quickly. A better plan is to increase your Level 2 activity: spend more time walking; cultivate a hobby that gets you moving; take up a sport instead of just watching. You'll burn extra calories and develop a healthier, more vibrant lifestyle. I really enjoy keeping active because it makes me feel so good. So, in addition to my runs, I make a point of walking whenever possible.

How You'll Feel Along the Way

I urge you to keep exercise logs. They will help you stay on track, and later you'll enjoy re-reading your early entries and marveling at the improvements. If you've never been physically active before, here's what you can expect over the next ten weeks.

During Weeks 1 to 4

You'll begin aerobic activity by Week 3. Most women I work with see a difference almost immediately, especially if they've been sedentary. First, they feel good about themselves for starting to exercise. They experience a post-exercise lift, and often tell me they have more energy throughout the day and sleep better at night.

Because this programme starts so gradually, you probably won't experience muscle soreness unless you've been very inactive. When soreness occurs, it usually doesn't develop right away. Instead, you feel it the day after. This is normal; the discomfort should disappear in a day or two. Unless it's severe (which is extremely unlikely), just continue with your workouts. Be sure to warm up, cool down, and stretch, to help your muscles and heart adjust to the exercise.

Some women experience joint pain when they begin an exercise programme. This rarely means that they've injured themselves. Usually they're uncovering an existing problem that was masked by inactivity. If this happens to you, progress more slowly and work out at Level 2 intensity instead of Level 3. In a week or two—when you've become stronger from strength training and aerobic activity—you should be able to exercise without joint pain.

During Weeks 5 to 10

By now your workouts should be familiar and comfortable. Indeed, I hope they're so enjoyable that you miss them if you have to skip a session.

To maintain Level 3 effort, you've probably stepped up the pace—you're walking a little faster, pedalling your bike a little harder. And you're able to sustain this effort for a longer time. All this is evidence that your body is getting fitter.

If you weren't able to take the walking test at the beginning, perhaps you are ready for it now. If you took the test, retake it when you're halfway through the programme. I think you'll be surprised by the progress you've made.

At the End of Week 10

Congratulations! You're exercising 30 minutes a day, at least three days a week—which puts you in the most active quarter of women in the western world. Depending on where you started, your cardiovascular fitness has probably increased by 10 to 20 per cent. What's more, you've developed an exercise habit that will keep you fit. Take the walking test again if you can; if you took it before, compare your score with earlier results. I'm sure you'll be very proud to see how far your hard work has taken you.

What's next? You might want to try new activities, or you can stick with what you're doing. As you continue to get fitter, you'll need to adjust your pace to maintain Level 3 effort. Some women are willing to invest the time in longer workouts. That's fine—just be sure to increase gradually, adding no more than 5 minutes to each session in a week. For example: take at least three weeks to increase your workouts from 30 minutes to 45 minutes.

BECOMING A MORE ACTIVE PERSON

I've been discussing Level 3 exercise, but I also want to emphasise how important it is—for weight reduction, for your health, and for your emotional well being—to be more active throughout the day. Here are a few suggestions:

- ♦ **Use yourself for transportation.** Instead of taking the shuttle bus at work, I walk the eight blocks from the parking garage to my office. When I'm running errands on the weekend, I walk the 2.5 kilometres (1¹/₂ miles) to town rather than using the car. This doesn't take a lot of time—in fact, sometimes I actually save time by walking.

- ♦ **Adopt active hobbies.** Try new sports; go dancing; take up gardening.

- **Socialise on the move.** Instead of meeting a friend for lunch, take a walk together. Play active games with your family.

- **Cultivate inefficiency.** Labour-saving devices keep you from burning calories! Rake the leaves instead of using an electric blower; if you live in a house with stairs, make a point of going up and down as often as possible.

ACTIVITIES

The easiest way to develop an exercise habit is to select an activity that's readily available and that you enjoy (or at least consider tolerable). Some people—including me—love to get outdoors to exercise. They want to breathe fresh air; they want to go places and see the countryside. Others prefer indoor workouts, for different but equally valid reasons. They don't have to worry about the weather, traffic, or unsafe neighbourhoods, and they can use exercise machines, which help calibrate effort. Either way is fine. I suggest you focus on one or two activities during the first ten weeks.

To help you decide, I'll discuss popular options that are particularly well suited to beginners. The list is by no means complete. If you belong to a gym, you may have access to many exercise machines, not just the few I've described. Anything that allows you to work at the right intensity, while feeling comfortable and safe, is good to use—a fitness instructor at the gym can help you get started.

You may be surprised that my list doesn't include tennis, squash, volleyball, or other competitive sports. These are terrific, enjoyable activities; if you're already doing them, just continue. Otherwise I don't recommend them for your "daily bread" workouts at this point. First, most of these activities aren't available every day, which is so important when you're trying to establish an exercise habit. In addition, they require bursts of activity plus sudden side movements, which are hard on your body unless you're already fit. So get in shape first, and then get involved in sports.

WALKING

Walking is often called the ideal aerobic exercise—and for good reason. Most of your muscles, as well as your cardiovascular system, get a workout when you walk. Walking tones your leg muscles. It's also great for weight control: it can use up a lot of calories, and it helps burn fat in the abdominal area.

If you walk outdoors, there's no need to purchase special equipment other than good shoes. Just be conscious of the outside temperature, and make sure your clothing is appropriate. An added convenience: you can tuck walking into your everyday routine, so you don't need to set aside much extra time for exercise.

Maintain good posture and swing your arms comfortably. As you become fitter, you'll need to increase intensity to maintain Level 3 effort. One way to do this is to walk faster. But once you reach 5 to 6.5 kilometres (3 to 4 miles) per hour—a very brisk walk—you'd have to jog or run, which is harder on your joints. If you want to break into a jog or run, I suggest you wait until you've been exercising for at least ten weeks; this reduces the risk of orthopaedic problems. In the meantime, you can reach Level 3 effort by walking uphill.

Some women increase intensity by carrying dumbbells or wearing wrist weights when they walk. If you've done this and feel you benefit, you can continue. But I don't recommend it. Adding weight can throw off your gait and balance, which could lead to joint problems. I think it's better to increase effort by going uphill or moving faster.

For those who'd rather walk indoors, treadmills are very popular. Use an electric treadmill rather than the kind powered by your movement. (Non-electric treadmills are more difficult to start and walk on, so it's harder to get a good workout. Also, they can be unsteady.) Look for a treadmill that's easy to adjust. The belt should be wide for you to feel steady when you walk. Make sure the walking surface is long enough for your stride, even if you move forward or back a little. Also important for safety are handrails on the side or front.

The first few times you use a treadmill, you may feel unsteady even if you don't normally have problems with balance. I suggest you gently hold on to the handrail until you're more comfortable. But as soon as you're able, try to walk without holding on because you'll have a better workout and burn more calories. Swing your arms and stride as you would if you were walking on the ground, with your heel striking the ground first. If you work out at a gym, ask a fitness instructor to check your form. To help maintain balance, find a focal point—something to look at that's straight ahead and about 3 to 6 metres (10 to 20 feet) away. If you need to turn your head, don't just spin around; hold the handrail and turn slowly.

As you lose weight and become fitter, you may find that you no longer reach Level 3 intensity. Adjustments are simple on the treadmill, since you can set the speed and incline. Try both kinds of increases to see which you prefer. However, during the first ten weeks, don't use an incline above 5 per cent.

Some treadmills (and other exercise machines) have built-in programmes that simulate walks over hilly terrain. While this feature is fun to use and adds variety to your workout, it may force you to work at an intensity that's too high or too low. Therefore, I suggest you stick with a fixed intensity for the first few weeks. After you're fitter you can experiment with different programmes.

CYCLING

Bike-riding and stationary cycling are also excellent exercises. Pedalling burns a lot of calories, and it works the muscles in your lower body. Cycling is great for your abdomen and it firms your bottom. Another important advantage is that it's easy on your joints. Also, many women find aerobic activity more enjoyable when they can do it sitting down. Cycling is a great way to have fun and go places—and it's something to do with others.

Stationary cycles come in different forms: upright, like an ordinary bicycle; or semi-recumbent, with a back to lean on for support. Most cycles train only the lower body, but some include an arm element that works the upper body. You might find those a bit difficult to use at first, since they require extra coordination. If so, start on a regular stationary cycle and focus on giving your legs a good workout.

When you buy a bicycle or stationary cycle, ask the sales person (or fitness instructor if you're at a gym) to help you get a good fit. The handlebars should be a comfortable distance in front, so your arms are neither cramped nor stretched out. Proper seat adjustment is also important for comfort. Adjust the height so that when your foot is flat on the pedal and the pedal is pushed all the way down, your knee is just slightly bent. You should feel comfortably balanced on the seat—experiment with the pitch, tilting it slightly forward or back, until you find a good position.

If you're using a stationary cycle, set the resistance so you can pedal at a rate of 55 to 65 revolutions per minute. As with the treadmill, I don't recommend using the built-in programmes that simulate hills until you've been exercising for several weeks. Two safety precautions: select clothing that won't get caught in the gears or wheels, and if you ride outdoors, always wear a helmet.

CROSS-COUNTRY SKIING

Cross-country skiing is an ideal aerobic exercise. It trains major muscles in the upper and lower body, and doesn't put a lot of strain on the joints. The entire trunk of your body—back, abdomen, and shoulders—will be firmer. Once you learn the move—and it can be tricky at first—you'll find cross-country skiing as easy as walking. Unfortunately, we don't live in locations that allow this to be our "daily bread" activity but cross-country skiing exercise machines have been developed to simulate the movements.

Ski machines are getting better and better. If you tried one a long time ago and didn't like it, give them another chance. Look for a machine that lets you adjust leg and arm resistance independently; some also let you increase the slope. With a little experimenting, you'll find the right settings.

Expect to spend a few sessions learning how to work the skis. It might help to hold on to the handles and do just the leg move at first. When you've mastered that, add the arm motion.

ROWING

Like cross-country skiing, rowing works your upper and lower body (including your abdomen)—but it doesn't put weight on your joints. This is another superb exercise that's more practical for most of us in its simulated form.

When you select a machine, check that the seat and "oars" (the bar you pull back) move very smoothly. I much prefer flywheel rowers to the hydraulic piston variety; I find the movement much smoother and more like real rowing. For safety, make sure the flywheel is encased.

The resistance and the stroke rate needn't be high to give you a great workout. Aim for 26 to 30 strokes per minute. Each stroke has two parts. First, you pull the oars towards your body and stretch out your legs to push the seat away from the flywheel, making sure not to lock your knees. Second, stretch your arms forwards, and bend your knees to bring the seat back towards the flywheel; your arms need to go past your knees before they bend. Try to make the movement smooth and fluid.

STAIR CLIMBING

Stair climbing is a terrific aerobic activity that some people—including me—find easy to fit into their lives. My office is on the fourteenth floor of a high-rise building. At least a couple of times a week, I make a point of using the stairs instead of the elevator. This isn't my "daily bread" activity, because it takes just five minutes. But it's a terrific stress-reducer.

Some athletes do stair-climbing workouts in outdoor stadiums, but for most people a stair-climbing machine is more practical. This very popular device provides great aerobic exercise, and it conditions the lower legs, abdomen, back, thighs, and calves. But stair climbers are not for everyone. If you have bad knees and can't comfortably use a regular stair climber, try a semi-recumbent model, which supports your body weight as you work out. Also, since stair climbers can elevate your heart rate very quickly, especially if you're heavy, progress gradually if you're out of shape.

Select a model that has a very smooth stepping action. The foot plates should be wide and secure enough to hold your foot steady without wobbling, and the handlebars should be easy to hold. Take natural steps; the ankle of your "up" foot should be between the calf and knee of your "down" foot; this generally means about 20 to 25 centimetres (8 to 10 inches).

Good posture is important. Stand tall and hold the rails lightly, just for balance. A common mistake is to grip the handrails and lean on them for support. But if you do that, your legs are not getting a full workout. If you can't keep up the pace in good form, that's a sign that you need to go more slowly or ease the resistance a bit.

CLASSES AND VIDEOS

Aerobics classes are a delightful way to work out. The moves can involve everything from dancing to boxing; some classes use equipment, including steps and weights. You may find a "spinning" class in which a trainer leads the group on a simulated bike ride through the country.

Talk with the instructor before you select a class. Make sure the required fitness level is appropriate for you—not too demanding, but sufficiently challenging so you'll have a Level 3 workout. For instance, step aerobics can be overly strenuous if you're out of shape or have knee problems. Chose a low-impact workout, where one foot is on the floor at all times, since this greatly lowers the risk of joint injuries. The class should include periods for warm-up, cool-down, and stretching.

What about "toning" aerobics classes that use light weights? They're fine if the aerobic intensity level is right for you. Just realise that you're only working your cardiovascular system; light weights will *not* increase your strength.

Exercise videos let you bring some of the fun of an aerobics class into your home. Read the box carefully to get the information an instructor would have provided. If possible, rent a video before you buy, to make sure it's appropriate and enjoyable.

SWIMMING AND AQUA AEROBICS

Swimming is an excellent exercise. You get an aerobic workout and also train major muscles in your upper and lower body. It's particularly appropriate for women with arthritis or orthopaedic problems, since your weight is supported by water. Learn different strokes—freestyle, breaststroke, and backstroke—to vary your routine and strengthen different muscles. Just be aware that it's a little harder to gauge intensity when you're in the water since you're not sweating, so learn to take your pulse.

Another popular water activity is aqua-aerobics. Led by a well-trained instructor, you can get an excellent, enjoyable workout that's easy on your joints because the water helps support your weight. Sometimes when I suggest aqua-aerobics, an overweight woman will confess that she feels self-conscious about putting on a bathing suit. But most classes have a wider range of body types than you'd expect, and participants have a great time once they're in the water.

9

A LIFELONG PLAN
FOR EATING WELL

I used to count calories rather than look at the kind of food I was eating. My diet didn't add up to good nutrition. I wasn't losing weight, even though I was skipping meals. I've cut down on portions. I'm aware when I've had enough protein and when I need to eat something with calcium. If I'm hungry, I have some fruit or a vegetable. Over six months I've lost 8 kilos (17 lb). It hasn't been that difficult because I have had plenty to eat.
—Nancy

◆   ◆   ◆

The *Strong Women Stay Slim* food plan is not a temporary diet that you'll force yourself to endure for a few months, then abandon with enormous relief after you lose weight. This plan will become a valuable part of your life. It's based on the US Food Guide Pyramid, which (as mentioned earlier) represents the best up-to-the-minute information from leading experts on nutrition and health, and has very similar British equivalents. I've used it with dozens of women—not only the volunteers in my research projects, but also friends and relatives who want to lose weight. I can assure you that it really works. The plan is health-promoting, flexible, and practical. You can follow it if you're travelling and eating in restaurants, if you're a vegetarian, if you have food allergies, or if you observe religious dietary restrictions.

Losing weight is just one of the benefits. Women who haven't been eating well are astonished by how good they feel when they're well nourished. They're more energetic and alert throughout the day. Gone are the sluggishness and the cranky low periods. Best of all, they're so pleased and proud of what they're doing for themselves.

THE POWER OF POSITIVE EATING

This food plan emphasises what you *should* eat, not what you *shouldn't* eat. Because good nutrition is so important, it's as much a mistake to skip a meal or omit a fruit as it is to have extra dessert.

TAKE TIME TO ENJOY

Eating good food is one of the great pleasures of life, so take the time to sit down and savour your meals. I realise this can be a challenge. If you're running errands at lunchtime, it's tempting to grab a sandwich and eat in the car. And many a weary mother has made an evening meal of her children's leftovers, consumed as she carries their plates from the table to the kitchen sink. But the time invested in preparing a wholesome dinner, setting the table, relaxing, and eating slowly really pays off. You'll find your meals much more satisfying, and that will help you stick with the food plan.

EAT WHATEVER YOU WANT— IN REASONABLE QUANTITY

There are no forbidden foods on this plan. You can have breads, pasta, eggs, red meat—and even butter, ice cream, and chocolate. After all, people who are naturally thin eat these foods. Of course, you'll have to limit the amount if you want to lose weight. But if you eat slowly, and concentrate on enjoying each mouthful, a modest serving can be very satisfying.

COUNT PORTIONS, NOT CALORIES

On this plan, you'll keep track of portions and types of food—dairy, grain, fruit, and so on—not calories. I prefer this system for two reasons. First, it's easy to use. You won't have to remember lots of details. Second, it promotes variety, a key to a healthy, well-balanced diet.

Note that I'm *not* saying that calories don't count—they definitely do! I'll refer to calories occasionally in this chapter; you may need to check calories if you want to add a food I haven't listed. But most of the time, you don't have to think about calories. If you follow the plan, you'll automatically be eating the correct number.

FIVE SIMPLE RULES THAT MINIMISE HUNGER AND MAXIMISE ENERGY

When you're well nourished—when your body has enough food and all the nutrients it needs—it's easier to lose weight. Your appetite is satisfied, so you are not derailed by hunger and cravings. You have energy throughout the day. Finally, you can get off the blood sugar roller coaster that leaves you desperate and irritable at some times, and groggy and bloated at others.

Here are five rules that optimise the nutritional payoff when you're following this food plan.

#1: EAT AT LEAST THREE MEALS A DAY

Your body and mind perform best with a steady supply of food. I often see a vicious circle that starts when a woman doesn't take time for breakfast. On the way to work she gulps a cup of coffee—she's kick-starting her engine, but she hasn't given it any fuel. Things get worse because she's too busy for lunch. By late afternoon, she's been fasting for twenty hours. Not surprisingly, she's ravenous and has trouble thinking clearly. She figures that since she hasn't eaten all day, she doesn't have to limit herself now. So on the way home she picks up a takeaway dinner that's high on fat but low on other nutrients. The next morning, still feeling the effects of the night before, she skips breakfast—and the whole situation repeats itself.

I strongly recommend that you eat three meals a day. You can also have one or more snacks, as you prefer. Some women get hungry between meals; for them, two or three snacks work well. Other women find that snacks actually make them hungrier, so they eat just at mealtime. I never get hungry between meals when I'm at work, but I like to have a snack when I get home, to take the edge off my hunger as I prepare dinner.

♦ ♦ ♦

I was a reckless, chaotic eater. I never planned. Some days I didn't eat anything until 3:30 in the afternoon. I was hungry without realising it. It was important for me to stabilise my eating and develop a regular meal plan.
— *Dianne*

♦ ♦ ♦

Sometimes women who are planning a special event ask me if they can "bank" calories—eat less than their daily plan permits for several days, so they can splurge later on. This is something I don't advise. Your body is working all the time, and it needs food to function optimally. You're much less likely to overeat at a special event if you've been well nourished throughout the week. If you arrive semi-starved, you'll find it more difficult to stay in control.

#2: INCLUDE AT LEAST THREE FOOD GROUPS AT EVERY MEAL

Your body needs carbohydrates and protein, and there's some evidence that your energy improves if you consume them together. Though this hasn't been extensively researched, my experience and that of other dietitians would suggest that people perform better if they eat a variety of foods throughout the day. Variety also makes for more interesting and satisfying meals. For instance, your sliced chicken sandwich will seem more like a complete lunch if you also have a piece of fruit. You may not be able to include three food groups at every meal, but I encourage you to try, especially at your main meal of the day.

#3: GO FOR A RAINBOW OF FRUITS AND VEGETABLES

Fruits and vegetables are low in calories and high in nutrients, which makes them ideal foods for weight loss. Nature has colour-coded them. For example, dark green vegetables are rich in calcium and folate; orange vegetables contain carotene, which your body converts to vitamin A. Therefore, a simple way to ensure that you're getting a healthy variety of nutrients is to enjoy an attractive mix of colours.

♦ ♦ ♦

I used to serve one vegetable with dinner; now I usually serve three. One of my favourite combinations in the winter is steamed broccoli, baked buttercup squash, and red cabbage. The colours are beautiful: green, bright orange, and deep purple. If there were just one vegetable, I wouldn't eat three portions. But if there's a variety, I do. This makes the meal much more filling. It's not a lot of work, because I choose vegetables that are simple to prepare, or I buy them ready-to-cook from the supermarket.
—Sarah

♦ ♦ ♦

#4: SELECT WHOLE GRAINS

Try to consume at least half of the day's grains in unprocessed form— whole wheat bread instead of white bread, brown rice instead of white. After grains are processed, manufacturers enrich them in an effort to restore lost nutrients. However, the enriched versions contain very little fibre, trace minerals, and other components of whole grains. Because of their fibre content, whole grains are digested more slowly than processed versions, so they keep your appetite satisfied longer.

#5: DRINK PLENTY OF FLUIDS

Your body needs to be well hydrated to function at its best. Most people are chronically under-hydrated because they don't drink enough. This is often an unsuspected factor in lethargy, fatigue, dry skin, and constipation. You may be surprised at how much better you look and feel when you start drinking more. Also, fluid is one of the great weight-loss aids. Sipping a beverage along with a meal or snack will help you feel satisfied sooner. Liquids also improve the performance of your digestive and metabolic systems.

Try to drink at least 2 litres (4 pints) of fluids a day, especially water.

A SIMPLE PRECAUTION

If you're following this plan for slow weight loss or to maintain your weight, you're probably getting all the nutrients you need. Still, just as a precaution, you might consider taking a multivitamin and mineral supplement.

However, most standard supplements contain much more than 100 per cent of the RDA (Recommended Daily Allowance) for the essential vitamins and minerals. Check the label to make sure the supplement supplies vitamin E, as well as folate and calcium— these are the nutrients many people miss in their diets, even if they eat well. If your multivitamin doesn't include calcium, consider a daily calcium supplement that contains 300 milligrams (if you're premenopausal) to 500 milligrams (if you're postmenopausal) or 600 milligrams (if you're breastfeeding); this will complement the calcium in your diet. Note: another option is to get extra nutrients from fortified foods, such as vitamin-fortified breakfast cereals or orange juice with added calcium.

Alcoholic and caffeinated beverages don't count because they stimulate the kidneys to increase urine volume, a dehydrating effect.

YOU CAN EAT MORE THAN YOU THOUGHT YOU COULD— AND STILL LOSE WEIGHT

The healthiest way to lose weight—and the best way to establish habits that will keep it off—is to eat a well-balanced diet that trims calories just enough to let you lose half to one kilogram (1 to 2 lb) a week. Many diet books put all women on 1000 to 1200 calories per day, no matter how active they are and no matter how much they weigh. But if you're doing strength training and aerobic exercise, you may be able to lose weight on 1500 to 2000 calories a day.

WHICH LEVEL IS RIGHT FOR YOU?

You've already learned how to adjust your exercise sessions so you gradually progress toward fitness goals. In the same way, you'll calibrate your food consumption so you lose between half to one kilogram (1 to 2 lb) per week. If you find you're losing too quickly, you'll eat a little more; if you're losing too slowly, you'll have a little less. After you reach your weight goal, similar adjustments will maintain your weight—and you'll know exactly how to make them.

For simplicity, I've included detailed information for three daily calorie levels: 1200, 1600 and 2000. Over time, you'll probably follow more than one of these plans.

HOW TO FIND YOUR STARTING POINT

The best way to determine a good starting point—what you'd do if you were working individually with a dietitian—is to keep a food diary for a week to find out how many calories you're consuming now. You'd then aim for a food plan that provides about 475 calories per day less than what you usually eat. This would let you lose half to one kilogram a week if you're also exercising.

IF YOUR GOAL IS	THIS IS YOUR PRELIMINARY STARTING LEVEL
To lose up to 10 kg (22 lb)	1600 calories
To lose 10 kg (22 lb) or more	1600 or 2000 calories
To maintain your current weight, but improve your eating habits	2000 calories

While you could do similar calculations on your own, most women can use the simple table on this page to arrive at an appropriate starting point.

Two exceptions:

♦ If you are already very physically active, start at 2000 calories even if you plan to lose less than 10 kilograms (22 lb).

♦ If you've been following a very stringent diet that provides much less food than the *Strong Women Stay Slim* plan recommends, and your weight is currently stable, decrease to the next lower calorie level—from 2000 to 1600, or from 1600 to 1200.

Don't worry if you're uncertain which level is best—this is just the beginning. Once you're following the plan and see how it works, you can easily adjust as needed.

THREE DAILY PLANS

The chart lists types of food and suggests the number of daily portions for three different calorie levels: 1200, 1600, and 2000. Following the chart are lists of specific foods, so you'll know how much a portion is.

The calorie counts are merely averages. One woman who meticulously follows the 1600-calorie plan may wind up eating closer to 1500 calories, because she happens to select lower-calorie items from the food list; another, just as careful, might consume nearly 1650 calories because her choices are consistently at the top of the range.

THE DAILY FOOD PLANS

FOOD GROUP	NUMBER OF PORTIONS EACH DAY		
	1200 CAL	1600 CAL	2000 CAL
Dairy: milk, yoghurt, cheese, soy equivalents	2	3	3
Protein: meat, poultry, fish, beans, tofu, eggs, nuts	4	5	6
Grain: bread, cereal, rice, pasta	5	6	8
Vegetable	3	4	5
Fruit	2	3	4
Extras: fats, oils, sweets	4	6	8

WHAT IS A PORTION?

'll use the word **portion** to mean a prescribed amount of a particular food. As you'll see, it's often not the amount you'd think of as a normal **serving**, which is the amount you'd put on your plate. For example, one portion of pasta is just half a 100g (4-oz). If you have pasta for dinner, your serving might be two or three Grain portions. A 125-gram (4-oz) serving of boneless chicken counts as four Protein portions.

Some items count as more than one food group. For example, a roast beef sandwich made from two slices of bread and 60 grams (2 oz) of roast beef would be two Grains for the bread and two Proteins for the meat.

Certain foods are higher in sugar or fat, so they contain more calories per portion than typical for their group. To compensate, these items draw upon your allotment of Extras. For example, if you have 275 ml (½ pint) of low-fat yoghurt, that counts as a Dairy portion plus 1 Extra; if you have a 125-gram (4-oz) pork chop, that's 4 Proteins plus 2 Extras. I've tried to list most common foods, but some of your favourites may be missing. If you can obtain calorie information (for instance, by reading a food label), you can work out portion equivalents.

PORTIONS OR CALORIES?

One reason I prefer to count portions rather than caloriesis that outside the laboratory, it's really impossible to determine calories precisely. I'm always amused when I see overly precise calories counts—like "453 calories per serving" on a recipe for vegetable lasagne. Was the grated cheese densely or loosely packed? Were all the servings cut exactly the same size or were some a centimetre wider than others? In reality, that "453 calories" lasagne serving could contain anywhere from around 380 to 500 or more calories.

When you start using the food plan, you'll need to check the lists frequently and the calculations may seem complex. But I promise you that in a week or two everything will be much easier. The Portion Primer that starts on page 195 will be very helpful.

Dairy (or Equivalents)

Dairy foods are very rich in high-quality protein, calcium (which is especially important for women), vitamin D (in the case of milk), riboflavin, and other vitamins and minerals. But most dairy products are also naturally high in saturated fat. Fortunately, there are excellent low-fat versions. If you use them, you won't miss out on any nutrients. In fact, a portion of skimmed milk actually has a little more calcium than whole milk. If you prefer soy milk, check the label to make sure it's fortified with calcium.

A dairy portion contains 90 to 120 calories. If you select a dairy food that's high in fat, such as ice cream or whole milk, you'll count the food as a Dairy portion plus 2 Extra portions; low-fat dairy foods count as a Dairy plus 1 Extra.

Milk, whole	275 ml (½ pint) (plus 2 Extras)
Milk, 1 to 2 per cent fat	275 ml (½ pint) (plus 1 Extra)
Milk, skimmed	275 ml (½ pint)
Soy or rice milk, with fat	275 ml (½ pint) (plus 1 Extra)
Soy or rice milk, non-fat	275 ml (½ pint)
Yoghurt, whole milk (plain or flavoured)	275 ml (½ pint) (plus 2 Extras)
Yoghurt, low-fat	275 ml (½ pint) (plus 1 Extra)
Yoghurt, skimmed	275 ml (½ pint)
Cottage cheese, whole milk	50 g (2 oz) (plus 2 Extras)
Cottage cheese, low-fat	50 g (2 oz) (plus 1 Extra)
Ricotta cheese, whole milk	60 g (2 oz) (plus 2 Extras)
Ricotta cheese, part skimmed	60 g (2 oz) (plus 1 Extra)
Hard cheese (Cheddar, Swiss)	30 g (1 oz) (plus 1 Extra)
Hard cheese, low-fat	30 g (1 oz)
Ice cream, regular	135 ml (¼ pint) (plus 2 Extras)
Ice cream, low-fat	135 ml (¼ pint) (plus 1 Extra)
Frozen yoghurt, low-fat	135 ml (¼ pint) (plus 1 Extra)
Dairy dessert, low-fat	135 ml (¼ pint) (plus 1 Extra)

PROTEIN

Meat, poultry, fish, beans, eggs, tofu, and nuts are important sources of protein, iron (especially red meat), zinc and several B vitamins. Like dairy foods, meats naturally contain fat. Therefore, it's best to choose the leanest cuts and to prepare them with as little added fat as possible. Notice that portions of most fish and tofu are twice as large as a portion of even lean meat or poultry. I encourage you to try tofu. As I mentioned in Chapter 4, soy products offer very important health benefits for women.

Each Protein portion contains 45 to 90 calories. If you select higher-fat foods, you'll have to compensate by cutting back your Extras.

Poultry, light meat without skin	25 g (1 oz)
Poultry, light meat with skin	25 g (1 oz) (plus ½ Extra)
Poultry, dark meat without skin	25 g (1 oz) (plus ½ Extra)
Poultry, dark meat with skin	25 g (1 oz) (plus 1 Extra)
Beef, lean (round, loin, flank)	25 g (1 oz)
Beef (chuck, hamburger)	25 g (1 oz) (plus ½ Extra)
Pork, lean (tenderloin, round)	25 g (1 oz)
Pork (chops, spareribs)	25 g (1 oz) (plus ½ Extra)
Lamb, lean (leg)	25 g (1 oz)
Lamb (chops)	25 g (1 oz) (plus ½ Extra)
Processed meat or poultry, low-fat	25 g (1 oz)
Processed meat, regular	25 g (1 oz) (plus ½ Extra)
Fish, light-coloured (flounder, flake)	60 g (2 oz)
Fish, dark-coloured (salmon, tuna)	30 g (1 oz)
Seafood (prawns, scallops)	60 g (2 oz)
Cooked legumes (kidney, lima, lentils, chickpeas)	100 g (4 oz)
Hummus (chickpea spread)	2 tablespoons
Egg	1 (plus 1 Extra)
Egg whites	3
Tofu	60 g (2 oz)
Nuts	30 g (1 oz) (plus 1 Extra)
Peanut butter	1 tablespoon (plus 2 Extras)

Grains

Grains, especially whole grains, are indeed the staff of life—the foundation of your diet. These foods are rich in B vitamins, minerals, complex carbohydrates, and fibre. Along with fruits and vegetables, they make your meals more enjoyable and filling.

Try to select unprocessed whole grains for at least half of your Grain allotment—brown rice, oats, barley, cracked wheat. If you're buying bread, look for "whole wheat flour" on the label. Don't assume that peasant-style loaves or "wheat flour" breads are made from whole grains. Often they're prepared with white flour to which molasses or a small amount of whole wheat flour has been added for colour.

Each Grain portion has 60 to 100 calories. Note that some ready-to-eat cereals contain added fat and sugar. Though these can be reasonable choices, especially as substitutes for sweet biscuits or cake—they count as Extras as well as Grains.

Bread	1 slice (30 g/1 oz)
Pitta	(30 g/1 oz) (1 very small or ½ of a regular round)
Bagel	½ small bagel (30 g/1 oz)
English muffin	½
Dinner roll	1 small (30 g/1 oz)
Cooked rice	100 g (4 oz)
Cooked pasta	100 g (4 oz)
Dry biscuits	5
Croutons	50 g (2 oz)
Chips, low-fat	30 g (1 oz)
Popcorn, no-fat	75 g (3 oz)
Rice cakes	2
Cooked cereal	100 g (4 oz)
Cold cereal, unsweetened	30 g (1 oz)
Cold cereal, lightly sweetened	30 g (1 oz) (plus 1 Extra)
Cold cereal, sweetened	30 g (1 oz) (plus 2 Extras)
Muesli	50 g (2 oz)

VEGETABLES

Vegetables provide many vitamins, minerals, health-promoting phytochemicals, and fibre. Most are naturally low in fat and calories. Consume a variety of vegetables to get nature's own multivitamin. Each vegetable portion contains approximately 10 to 40 calories—the lowest of all the food groups.

Cooked green vegetables, carrots, courgettes, aubergine, mushrooms, red cabbage, cauliflower	50 g (2 oz)
Lettuce, raw cabbage, or raw spinach	200 g (7 oz)
Sprouts	100 g (4 oz)
Raw vegetables, chopped or sliced	50 g (2 oz)
Artichoke	1/2 of medium artichoke
Asparagus	6 spears
Avocado	35 g (1 oz) (plus 2 Extras)
Brussels sprouts	4 cooked
Carrot	1 medium; 6 baby carrots
Celery stalks	4
Sweetcorn	1/2 ear; 25 g (1 oz) kernels
Peas	25 g (1 oz)
Tomato	1 whole; 75 g (3 oz) chopped
Onion	1 whole; 75 g (3 oz) chopped
Potato, baked with skin	1/2 small potato
Potato, mashed (include Extras if mashed with butter or soured cream)	35 g (1 oz)
Sweet potato with skin	1/2 small potato
Vegetable juice	185 ml (1/3 pint)
Vegetable soup	250 ml (1/2 pint)
Tomato sauce	125 ml (1/4 pint)

FRUITS

Luscious fruits, along with vegetables, contribute numerous vitamins, minerals, and phytochemicals to your diet. Citrus fruits are especially good sources of vitamin C; they also contain some calcium. In addition, the fibre in fruit fills you up and keeps your digestive system moving. As you cut back on empty-calorie desserts and snacks, you'll find the sweetness of fruit more satisfying. A portion of fruit contains 80 to 100 calories.

Fruit (apple, orange, kiwifruit, peach, nectarine)	1 medium
Fresh fruit, diced	75 g (3 oz)
Fruit, canned in unsweetened juice	75 g (3 oz)
Fruit, canned in sweetened juice	75 g (3 oz) (plus 1 Extra)
Fruit juice (100% juice)	250 ml (½ pint)
Banana	1 small
Grapefruit	½
Plums	2
Apricots	4
Figs	2
Mango	½
Melon, diced	200 g (7 oz)
Berries, cherries, grapes	75 g (3 oz)
Coconut, fresh	50 by 50 by 15 mm piece (plus 2 Extras)
Coconut, dry	30 g (1 oz) (plus 2 Extras)
Dried fruit	50 g (2 oz)
Dried apple rings	4
Raisins/sultanas	2 tablespoons

EXTRAS

The list of foods in this category may surprise you since it includes butter, oil, whipped cream, confectionary, sugar, and other items that many diet plans exclude. Most dietitians would not consider them a food group, but I'm adding them for several reasons.

First, as you've already seen, this category helps you keep track when you select higher-calorie options from the other groups. For instance, a glass of whole milk counts as 1 Dairy portion plus 2 Extras. Added fat is also in this category. In limited quantity, fat is actually useful when you're trying to lose weight. It carries flavour, and because it's broken down more slowly than protein or carbohydrate, fat helps you feel full longer after a meal. Similarly, controlled amounts of sugar can make your food plan more flexible and appealing. And, of course, many people enjoy alcoholic beverages. (Some research suggests that the flavonoids in red wine are health-promoting.)

Vegetable and olive oil	1 teaspoon
Butter, margarine, regular mayonnaise (use sparingly because of saturated fats and trans fatty acids)	1 teaspoon
Diet margarine	2 teaspoons
Cream cheese, regular	1 tablespoon
Cream cheese, low-fat	2 tablespoons
Cream, whipped	1 tablespoon
Sour cream, standard	1 tablespoon
Sour cream, low-fat	2 tablespoons
Salad dressing, standard	2 teaspoons
Salad dressing, low-fat	4 teaspoons
Sugar, brown sugar, honey, sweet syrup, jam, chocolate syrup	2 teaspoons
Muesli bar	½ bar
Hard confectionery, cough drop	3
Sweet biscuit, 3–5 cm (1–2 in) in diameter	1
Crackers	3
Crisps, fried (potato, etc.)	10 g (½ oz) (about 5 crisps)
Fried chips	25 g (1 oz) (about 5 chips)
Soft drink	250 ml (½ pint)
Beer, standard	250 ml (½ pint)
Beer, light	500 ml (1 pint)
Wine	250 ml (½ pint)
Spirits (gin, vodka, whisky, etc.)	30 ml (⅙ gill)
Sweet liqueur	15 ml (1/12 gill)

An Extra portion contains 30 to 70 calories Remember, some of your daily Extras may come from your selections in the other food groups.

WHAT ABOUT SOUPS, CASSEROLES, AND OTHER MULTI-INGREDIENT FOODS?

After a few weeks on this food plan, you'll be able to glance at a plate and know that it contains, say, about 90 grams (3 oz) of chicken (3 Proteins), 200 g (7 oz) of rice (2 Grains) and 50 g (2 oz) of sliced carrots (1 Vegetable). But suppose you're at a dinner party, and the hostess serves a seafood pasta casserole in a cheese sauce. How should you count your serving?

Short of requesting a recipe plus measuring utensils, all you can do is guess. Make a quick mental list of ingredients, then estimate portion sizes. For instance, you might figure that your serving of seafood casserole includes about 100 g (4 oz) of pasta (2 Grains) approximately 200 g (7 oz) of seafood (2 Proteins), some chopped vegetables (1 Vegetable), plus about 135 ml (½ pint) of creamy sauce (call it a ½ Dairy plus 2 Extras).

What if you're wrong? Provided you are not consistently underestimating your consumption, day after day, it really doesn't matter if you're slightly too high or too low at one meal. Do your best, then relax and enjoy the party.

Here are a few examples of combination foods:

Cheese pizza: ⅛ of 30-cm (12 in) size	1 Grain, 1.5 Dairy, 2 Extras
Salami pizza: ⅛ of 30-cm (12 in) size	1 Grain, 1.5 Dairy, 1 Protein, 3 Extras
Cheeseburger: 120g (4 oz) burger	2 Grains, 1 Dairy, 4 Proteins, 3 Extras
Macaroni cheese: 200g (7 oz)	2 Grains, 1.5 Dairy, 3 Extras
Fruit pie: ⅛ of 25-cm (10 in)	1 Fruit, 1 Grain, 3 Extras
Chocolate layer cake: 1/12 of 25-cm (10 in) (2-layer cake with frosting)	1 Grain, 4 Extras

THE NEXT-TO-NOTHING LIST

To simplify the plan and give you added flexibility, I've compiled a list of foods that are so low in calories, or used in such small quantities, that you don't have to count them. This means that when you're enjoying a roast beef sandwich topped with lettuce and tomato, seasoned with mustard, accompanied by a few dill pickle slices, and garnished with parsley—that's just two Grains for the roll and three Proteins for the beef.

The NTN list is also your insurance against hunger. Use it for snacks and to expand meals. Note: I called this list "*Next-to*-Nothing" for a reason. Most items on the list contain a few calories. So I want to caution you that you could undermine your efforts if you eat very large quantities—that's why I've placed daily limits on some items.

You may be puzzled to see some items on the NTN list that are also on the Vegetable list. These can be counted either way. For instance, if you're hungry and want more vegetables than your food plan calls for, have a plate of sliced cucumber, pepper and celery—and record the whole snack as NTN. But if you're behind on vegetables, and need another portion to reach your daily quota, you could count the same snack as a Vegetable.

Beverages

Water	Soda
Diet soft drink	Coffee
Soup, broth (250 ml (½ pint); may be high in salt)	Tea

Sauces, Seasonings, Garnishes, and Condiments

Garlic
Mustard
Fresh ginger
Horseradish
Soy sauce, teriyaki sauce
Hot sauce
Worcestershire sauce
Vinegar
Lemon juice, lime juice
Non-stick spray
Herbs and spices (basil, cinnamon, curry, dill, oregano, etc.)
Flavour extracts (vanilla, almond, etc.)
Fruit or vegetable garnishes (a few slices of onion, tomato, orange, etc.)

Dill pickle (1; high in salt)
Relish (1 tablespoon; high in salt)
Salsa made without oil (3 tablespoons; may be high in salt)
Tomato sauce (1 tablespoon; high in salt)
Barbecue sauce (1 tablespoon; high in salt)

VERY LOW-CALORIE RAW VEGETABLES

Lettuce	Radish
Spinach	Mushrooms
Cabbage	Celery
Sprouts	Green pepper
Cucumber	

VEGETABLES: THE SAFETY VALVE

When you're really hungry and need to supplement a meal or have a snack, reach for vegetables—especially the ones on the Next-to-Nothing list. They'll fill you up and satisfy the need to chew, while providing extra nutrients.

- ◆ Snack on crunchy raw veggies—celery, cucumber.
- ◆ Enlarge a meal with a generous serving of salad.
- ◆ Use vegetables to add bulk to sandwiches, soups, casseroles, stir-fries, and other dishes.

SUGAR-FREE SWEETS

Sugar-free hard confectionary or gum (limit to 5 pieces)
Sugar-free gelatine dessert (limit to 100 g (4 oz), prepared)

BAKING AND COOKING INGREDIENTS

Cocoa, unsweetened (up to 1 tablespoon)
Cornflour, flour, farina (up to 1 tablespoon)
Gelatine, dry unsweetened (up to 1 sachet)

THE PORTION PRIMER

One key to success in this plan is correct portion size. Have you ever wondered how most French women stay slim, despite the rich cream sauces and buttery pastries? Their secret is small servings. I recently attended an international nutrition conference in Paris, and went out for dinner with several French friends. By American standards, the servings were tiny. My main dish consisted of one small lamb chop, four slices of potato, and a small portion of slivered carrots; dessert was about two tablespoons of intensely flavoured lemon sorbet, served in a beautiful crystal glass. But these were just two courses in a six-course dinner. Because the servings were so small, I was able to sample a wide variety of foods—and afterwards I felt satisfied instead of uncomfortably stuffed. In the United States, restaurant servings are three times as large!

Almost always, if a woman tells me she's following the food plan and not losing weight, the culprit is portion size. She may not realise that her breakfast bagel is the equivalent of three or four Grain portions, or that her normal serving of yoghurt is two Dairy portions.

If you're following the plan and getting the results you want, you're probably using proper portions. But if you run into trouble, I urge you to spend a day or two familiarising yourself with correct portion size. You'll quickly learn how to estimate portions, and afterwards you won't need to weigh and measure. Here are a few tips:

- ◆ Use measuring cups to serve foods like rice, pasta, mashed potatoes, and soup.

- ◆ Fill a serving utensil with water, then measure to see how much it holds. For instance, I know that my ice cream scoop holds 70 ml (⅛ pint), and that my soup ladle holds a 135 ml (¼ pint).

- ◆ Notice how a portion looks in a bowl or on your plate. Thereafter you'll recognise 275 ml (½ pint) of soup or 300 g (11 oz) of pasta.

Large bread roll: 125 g (4 oz)

Medium bread roll: 90 g (3 oz)

Small bread roll: 60 g (2 oz)

Bread rolls and other bakery items often are larger than you might expect. In the beginning, I suggest you weigh the foods you use regularly to learn how many portions they contain—remember that 30 g (1 oz) equals 1 Grain. After a while, you'll become familiar with different sizes and you'll be able to estimate.

Large potato: 6 portions

Medium potato: 4 portions

Small potato: 2 portions

One Vegetable portion is just ½ of a small potato. A small potato is smaller than your fist.

All three of the servings above contain 1 portion of apple. It's interesting to see that when you dice or slice an apple, it looks as though there's more to eat.

All four of these servings contain 30 g (1 oz) of cheese.

Chicken: 120 g (4 oz)

Hamburger patty: 120 g (4 oz)

Sliced tofu: 250 g (9 oz)

Fish: 250 g (9 oz)

All of these servings are 4 Protein portions. Note that you get twice as much food if you eat fish or tofu. I've placed a deck of cards on the platter for reference, to help you learn how to estimate portions.

Most people don't realise how easy it is to have more pasta portions than they intend. The small serving is 100 g (4 oz) of cooked spaghetti, which is 1 Grain portion. The larger serving is twice as big—200 g (7 oz), or 2 Grains.

SAMPLE MENUS

When I work with a woman who's beginning to follow the food plan, we start by planning menus—meals and snacks—for one or two days. I ask her to write down her favourite foods, so we can make sure they're included. We also discuss any special circumstances that affect her food choices, such as her work schedule. I encourage you to do the same. Sit down with the book and a pad, and come up with a few menus. Most women find the planning process very helpful. They're delighted to see how easily the food plan fits into their life, and they're surprised at how much they can eat.

Below are five different menus, designed for five different women. As you'll see, their individual needs are readily accommodated. After you've been following the food plan for a while, you might welcome still more flexibility. In Chapter 12, I have a few suggestions that could be helpful.

♦ ♦ ♦

I lost the 5 kilos (11 lb) I wanted to lose, and I've kept it off for a year—but I still fill out my food chart every morning and plan my three meals. It helps me stay balanced. I decide what my extras will be—wine with dinner, or confectionary if that's what I'm craving. If I'm going out for an Italian dinner, I plan a breakfast and lunch without Grains so I can have a big serving of pasta at night. Being organised about what I'm eating is half the battle.
—Susan

♦ ♦ ♦

"I'm very busy; I don't have time to fuss"

This menu is for a working mum who likes to keep things simple in the morning. It includes a packed lunch and snacks for coffee breaks. A stir-fry made from supermarket vegetables provides the basis for a quick and easy dinner.

1200 CAL	1600 CAL	2000 CAL
Breakfast	**Breakfast**	**Breakfast**
Orange jce, 250 ml (¹/₂ pint) (1F)	Orange jce, 250 ml (¹/₂ pint)(1F)	Orange jce, 250 ml (¹/₂ pint(1F)
Cereal, 30 g (1 oz) (1G)	Cereal, 30 g (1 oz) (1G)	Cereal, 30 g (1 oz) (1G)
Skimmed milk, 275 ml (¹/₂ pint) (1D)	Skimmed milk, 275 ml (¹/₂ pint) (1D)	Skimmed milk, 275 ml (¹/₂ pint) (1D)
Sugar, 2 tsp (1E)	Sugar, 2 tsp (1E)	Sugar, 2 tsp (1E)
Snack	**Snack**	**Snack**
Sweet biscuit, 1 sm (1E)	Sweet biscuit, 1 sm (1E)	Sweet biscuit, 1 sm (1E)
Coffee, black	Coffee, black	Coffee, black
Lunch	**Lunch**	**Lunch**
Chicken sandwich:	Chicken-cheese sandwich:	Chicken-cheese sandwich:
Lean chicken,	Lean chicken,	Lean chicken, 120g (4 oz)(4P)
60g (2 oz)(2P)	90g (3 oz)(3P)	Low-fat cheese,
1 roll, 60g (2 oz) (2G)	Low-fat cheese,	30g (1 oz) (1D, 1E)
Mustard, lettuce,	30g (1 oz) (1D, 1E)	1 roll, 60g (2 oz) (2G)
tomato slice	1 roll, 60g (2 oz) (2G)	Mustard, lettuce, tomato slice
Baby carrots, 6 (1V)	Mustard, lettuce, tomato slice	Baby carrots, 12 (2V)
Diet cola	Baby carrots, 6 (1V)	Raisins, 4 tbsp (2F)
	Raisins, 2 tbsp (1F)	Diet cola
	Diet cola	
Snack	**Snack**	**Snack**
Pitta chips, 30g (1 oz)(1G)	Pitta chips, 30g (1 oz)(1G)	Pitta chips, 60g (2 oz)(2G)
Herbal tea	Herbal tea	Herbal tea

1200 CAL

Dinner

Prawn stir fry:

Oil, 2 tsp (2E)

Mixed vegetables,
100 g (4 oz) (2V)

Frozen prawns,
120g (4 oz) (2P)

Rice, 100 g (4 oz) (1G)

Low-fat yoghurt,
140 ml (¼ pint) (1D)

Frozen berries,
75 g (3 oz) (1F)

Totals

Dairy: 2

Protein: 4

Grain: 5

Vegetable: 3

Fruit: 2

Extras: 4

1600 CAL

Dinner

Prawn stir fry:

Oil, 3 tsp (3E)

Mixed vegetables,
300 g (11 oz) (3V)

Frozen prawn,
120g (4 oz) (2P)

Rice, 200 g (7 oz) (2G)

Low-fat yoghurt,
140 ml (¼ pint) (1D)

Frozen berries,
75 g (3 oz) (1F)

Totals

Dairy: 3

Protein: 5

Grain: 6

Vegetable: 4

Fruit: 3

Extras: 6

2000 CAL

Dinner

Prawn stir fry:

Oil, 3 tsp (3E)

Mixed vegetables,
300 g (11 oz) (3V)

Frozen prawns,
120g (4 oz) (2P)

Rice, 200 g (7 oz) (2G)

Low-fat yoghurt,
140 ml (¼ pint) (1D)

Frozen berries,
75 g (3 oz) (1F)

Whipped cream,
2 tbs (2E)

Totals

Dairy: 3

Protein: 6

Grain: 7

Vegetable: 5

Fruit: 4

Extras: 8

"I'm always hungry"

Appetite-appeasing features of this menu include three between-meal snacks, high-fibre choices, and items from the Next-to-Nothing list to round out meals.

1200 CAL	1600 CAL	2000 CAL
Breakfast	**Breakfast**	**Breakfast**
Orange, cut-up (1F)	Orange, cut-up (1F)	Orange, cut-up (1F)
Porridge, 50 g (2 oz) (1G)	Porridge, 50 g (2 oz) (1G)	Porridge, 100 g (4 oz) (2G)
Brown sugar, 1 tsp ($^1/_2$E)	Brown sugar, 2 tsp (1E)	Brown sugar, 4 tsp (2E)
Café latte ($^1/_2$D)	Café latte ($^1/_2$D)	Café latte ($^1/_2$D)
Snack	**Snack**	**Snack**
Cold cereal, 30 g (1 oz) (1G)	Cold cereal, 30 g (1 oz) (1G)	Cold cereal, 30 g (1 oz) (1G)
Milk, low-fat,	Milk, low-fat,	Milk, low-fat,
140 ml ($^1/_4$ pint) ($^1/_2$D)	140 ml ($^1/_4$ pint) (($^1/_2$D)	140 ml ($^1/_4$ pint) ($^1/_2$D)
Lunch	**Lunch**	**Lunch**
Broth, 250 ml ($^1/_2$ pint) (NTN)	Broth, 250 ml ($^1/_2$ pint) (NTN)	Broth, 250 ml ($^1/_2$ pint) (NTN)
Bean salad in pitta:	Bean salad in pitta:	Bean salad in pitta:
Pitta, 1 small (1G)	Pittas, 2 small (2G)	Pittas, 2 small (2G)
Chickpeas, 50 g (2 oz) (1P)	Chickpeas, 50 g (2 oz) (2P)	Chickpeas, 50 g (2 oz) (2P)
Tomato, onion, salsa (NTN)	Tomato, onion, salsa (NTN)	Tomato, onion, salsa (NTN)
Fruit-flavoured herbal tea	Melon, 150 g (5 oz) (1F)	Melon, 200 g (7 oz) (2F)
	Fruit-flavoured herbal tea	Fruit-flavoured herbal tea
Snack	**Snack**	**Snack**
Veggie munchies:	Veggie munchies:	Veggie munchies:
Green pepper strips, mushrooms, radishes, celery sticks (NTN)	Green pepper strips, mushrooms, radishes, celery sticks (NTN)	Green pepper strips, mushrooms, radishes, celery sticks (NTN)
Popcorn, plain, 75 g (3 oz) (1G)	Popcorn, plain, 75 g (3 oz) (1G)	Popcorn, plain, 150 g (5 oz) (2G)
Mineral water with lime	Mineral water with lime	Mineral water with lime

1200 CAL

Dinner

Salad:

  Lettuce, sprouts (NTN)

  Low-fat dressing,

  2 tsp (^{1}/2E)

Garlic bread (1G, 1E)

Flounder, 180g (6 oz)(3P)

Potato, small (2V)

Butter, 1 tsp (1E)

Broccoli, 50 g (2 oz) (1V)

Apple slices (1F)

Indian spice tea

Snack

Low-fat yoghurt,

140 ml (^{1}/4 pint) (1D, 1E)

Totals

Dairy: 2

Protein: 4

Grain: 5

Vegetable: 3

Fruit: 2

Extras: 4

1600 CAL

Dinner

Salad:

  Lettuce, sprouts (NTN)

  Low-fat dressing,

  4 tsp (1E)

Garlic bread (1G, 1E)

Flounder, 180g (6 oz)(3P)

Potato, small (2V)

Butter, 1 tsp (1E)

Broccoli,100 g (4 oz) (2V)

Apple slices (1F)

Indian spice tea

Snack

Low-fat yoghurt,

275 ml (^{1}/2 pint) (2D, 2E)

Totals

Dairy: 3

Protein: 5

Grain: 6

Vegetable: 4

Fruit: 3

Extras: 6

2000 CAL

Dinner

Salad:

  Lettuce, sprouts (NTN)

  Low-fat dressing,

  4 tsp (1E)

Garlic bread (1G, 1E)

Flounder, 200g (7oz)(4P)

Potato, medium (3V)

Butter, 2 tsp (2E)

Broccoli, 100 g (4 oz) (2V)

Apple slices (1F)

Indian spice tea

Snack

Low-fat yoghurt,

275 ml (^{1}/2 pint) (2D, 2E)

Totals

Dairy: 3

Protein: 6

Grain: 8

Vegetable: 5

Fruit: 4

Extras: 8

"I CRAVE SWEETS"

Judicious use of Extras helps satisfy a sweet tooth. And this menu includes generous mid-day snacks.

1200 CAL	1600 CAL	2000 CAL
Breakfat	**Breakfast**	**Breakfast**
Raisin bread, toasted (1G)	Raisin bread, toasted (1G)	Raisin bread, toasted (2G)
Ricotta, low-fat, 60g (2 oz) (1D)	Ricotta, low-fat, 120g (4 oz) (2D)	Ricotta, low-fat, 120g (4 oz) (2D)
Strawberries, 150 g (5oz) (1F)	Strawberries, 150 g (5 oz) (1F)	Strawberries, 150 g (5 oz) (1F)
Coffee	Coffee	Coffee
Snack	**Snack**	**Snack**
Cereal, lightly sweetened 30 g (1 oz) (1G, 1E)	Cereal, lightly sweetened 30 g (1 oz)(1G, 1E)	Cereal, lightly sweetened 60 g (2 oz)(2G, 2E)
Herbal tea, fruit flavour	Herbal tea, fruit flavour	Raisins, 2 tbsp (1F)
		Herbal tea, fruit flavour
Lunch	**Lunch**	**Lunch**
Hummus sandwich:	Hummus sandwich:	Hummus sandwich:
Wholegrain bread (2G)	Wholegrain bread (2G)	Wholegrain bread (2G)
Hummus, 2 tbsp (1P)	Hummus, 2 tbsp (1P)	Hummus, 4 tbsp (2P)
Lettuce, tomato slice (NTN)	Lettuce, tomato slice (NTN)	Lettuce, tomato slice (NTN)
Carrot sticks (1V)	Carrot sticks (1V)	Carrot sticks (2V)
Mineral water with lime	Mineral water with lime	Mineral water with lime
Small banana (1F)	Small banana (1F)	Small banana (1F)
Jelly babies 30 g (1 oz)(1E)	Jelly babies 30 g (1 oz)(1E)	Jelly babies 30 g (1 oz)(1E)
Snack	**Snack**	**Snack**
Chocolate milk shake:	Chocolate milk shake:	Chocolate milk shake:
Milk, skimmed, 275 ml (¹/₂ pint) (1D)	Milk, skimmed, 275 ml (¹/₂ pint) (1D	Milk, skimmed, 275 ml (¹/₂ pint) (1D)
Chocolate milkshake powder, (1E)	Chocolate milkshake powder, (2E)	Chocolate milkshake powder, (2E)
Ice cubes	Ice cubes	Ice cubes
		Crackers, 7 (1E)

1200 CAL

Dinner

$^1/_2$ warm pitta bread (1G)

Salsa (NTN)

Chicken breast, 90g (3 oz)(3P)

Small potato (2V)

Spinach (NTN)

Decaf espresso

1 glass wine (1E)

Totals

Dairy: 2

Protein: 4

Grain: 5

Vegetable: 3

Fruit: 2

Extras: 4

1600 CAL

Dinner

1 small warm pitta bread (2G)

Salsa (NTN)

Chicken breast,
120g (4 oz) (4P)

Medium potato (3V)

Spinach (NTN)

Decaf espresso

1 glass wine (1E)

Apple (1F)

Totals

Dairy: 3

Protein: 5

Grain: 6

Vegetable: 4

Fruit: 3

Extras: 5

2000 CAL

Dinner

1 warm pitta bread (2G)

Salsa (NTN)

Chicken breast,
120g (4 oz) (4P)

Medium potato (3V)

Spinach (NTN)

Decaf espresso

1 glass wine (1E)

Apple (1F)

Totals

Dairy: 3

Protein: 6

Grain: 8

Vegetable: 5

Fruit: 4

Extras: 7

"I'M A VEGETARIAN"

Only the Protein category contains meat, and vegetarians can select from a wide variety—eggs, beans, tofu, and nuts—on this food plan.

1200 CAL	1600 CAL	2000 CAL
Breakfast	**Breakfast**	**Breakfast**
Porridge, 50 g (2 oz) (1G)	Porridge, 50 g (2 oz) (1G)	Porridge, 100 g (4 oz) (2G)
Skimmed milk, 275 ml (¹/₂ pint) (1D)	Skimmed milk, 275 ml (¹/₂ pint) (1D)	Skimmed milk, 275 ml (¹/₂ pint) (1D)
Banana, sliced (1F)	Banana, sliced (1F)	Banana, sliced (1F)
Coffee	Sultanas, 2 tbsp (1F)	Sultanas, 2 tbsp (1F)
	Coffee	Coffee
Snack	**Snack**	**Snack**
Granny Smith apple (1F)	Granny Smith apple (1F)	Granny Smith apple (1F)
		Whole wheat toast,
		1 slice (1G)
		Peanut butter,
		1 tbsp (1P, 2E)
		Iced tea with lemon
Lunch	**Lunch**	**Lunch**
Veggie burger sandwich:	Veggie burger sandwich:	Veggie burger sandwich:
Veggie burger,	Veggie burger,	Veggie burger,
120g (4 oz) (2P)	120g (4 oz) (2P)	120g (4 oz) (2P)
Multigrain bun,	Multigrain bun,	Multigrain bun,
60g (2 oz) (2G)	60g (2 oz) (2G)	60g (2 oz)(2G)
Lettuce, tomato, onion	Cheddar cheese,	Cheddar cheese,
Spicy mustard	30g (1 oz) (1D, 1E)	30g (1 oz) (1D, 1E)
Baby carrots, 6 (1V)	Lettuce, tomato, onion	Lettuce, tomato, onion
Soda with lemon	Spicy mustard	Spicy mustard
	Baby carrots, 12 (2V)	Baby carrots, 12 (2V)
	Soda with lemon	Tomato juice,
		185 ml (¹/₃ pint) (1V)
Snack	**Snack**	**Snack**
Low-fat apricot yoghurt,	Low-fat apricot yoghurt,	Low-fat apricot yoghurt,
275 ml (¹/₂ pint) (1D, 1E)	275 ml (¹/₂ pint) (1D, 1E)	275 ml (¹/₂ pint) (1D, 1E)

1200 CAL

Dinner

Grilled firm tofu,
  120g (4 oz) (2P)

Grilled vegetables,
  100 g (4 oz) (2V)

prepared with:

Oil, 2 tsp (2E)

Teriyaki sauce, garlic, ginger

Brown rice, 200 g (7 oz) (2G)

Herbal tea

Crackers, 3 (1E)

Totals

Dairy: 2

Protein: 4

Grain: 5

Vegetable: 3

Fruit: 2

Extras: 4

1600 CAL

Dinner

Grilled firm tofu,
  180g (6 oz) (3P)

Grilled vegetables,
  100 g (4 oz) (2V)

prepared with:

Oil, 2 tsp (2E)

Teriyaki sauce, garlic, ginger

Brown rice,
  300 g (11 oz) (3G)

Herbal tea

Crackers, 6 (2E)

Totals

Dairy: 3

Protein: 5

Grain: 6

Vegetable: 4

Fruit: 3

Extras: 6

2000 CAL

Dinner

Sliced strawberries,
  200 g (7 oz)(1F)

Grilled firm tofu,
  180g (6 oz)(3P)

Grilled vegetables,
  100 g (4 oz) (2V)

prepared with:

Oil, 2 tsp (2E)

Teriyaki sauce, garlic, ginger

Brown rice,
  300 g (11 oz) (3G)

Herbal tea

Crackers, 6 (2E)

Totals

Dairy: 3

Protein: 6

Grain: 8

Vegetable: 5

Fruit: 4

Extras: 8

PULLING IT ALL
TOGETHER

When I'm following an exercise schedule, when I'm aware of what I'm eating and how much, I feel more in control, more confident, more powerful. And that creates a ripple effect in my life. I have more patience, I'm calmer, I'm more compassionate. When my eating is out of control and when I'm not doing any exercise, I feel that other aspects of my life are out of control.
    —Therese

◆ ◆ ◆

Each component of the *Strong Women Stay Slim* weight-loss programme—the strength-training exercises, the aerobic activities, and the food plan—is beneficial by itself. But they're also connected. As you bring the pieces together, you'll be pleased to discover how much they complement each other. Of course, your aerobic workouts become easier as you get stronger. Exercise, in turn, can help regulate your appetite. And a better diet gives you more energy for physical activity. Most important, as you make healthy changes for yourself and begin to see the resulting improvements, you'll have a wonderful sense of accomplishment that will make all your efforts easier.

Here's how to make it happen.

THE WEEK BEFORE YOU START

You've read Chapters 7, 8 and 9, which tell you how to do this programme, and you may be well on your way. Perhaps you've bought dumbbells, picked out an aerobic activity, and started to plan menus. If so, congratulations! But if you need a little help to get moving, I'd like to give you some suggestions.

SIT DOWN WITH THIS BOOK, A PAD, A PENCIL, AND YOUR CALENDAR

As you know by now, I'm a strong believer in the power of lists and appointments. Just writing things down helps you get organised. Then, as you start checking off items, the list becomes both stimulus and reward. If your life is crowded with obligations, putting a task on your calendar assures uninterrupted time to get it done.

I realise that some women don't like "to do" lists and appointment calendars. If you're among them, I recommend you give yourself a deadline for starting the programme. Later, if you find that the deadline has passed but you're still not up and running, please give this technique a try.

GET READY TO STRENGTH TRAIN

The strength-training programme requires dumbbells. If you don't have them already, reread pages 108–109 to learn what you'll need. Figure out

IF YOU SET A STARTING DATE

You may have seen the humorous T-shirt slogan: *Eat, drink and be merry, for tomorrow you diet.* But it's no joke when a woman overeats for five days in anticipation of starving to lose weight—and winds up feeling bloated and disgusted with herself.

Remember that there are no forbidden foods on this programme. There's no need to eat a desperate "last meal". If you don't want to begin right away, give yourself a positive head start by eating more fruits, vegetables, and whole grains.

HOW TO FIND A GYM

Check your Yellow Pages under "Health Clubs and Fitness Centres". There may be gyms at your local community centre, or at a nearby school. Convenience is a must. You'll find it much easier to go regularly if the facility is near your home or work and the hours match yours.

Ring the clubs you're considering, and arrange for a tour. If possible, visit at the same time you'd be there to work out. Here are things to look for and questions to ask:

- Is everything well lit and clean? (Use your nose as well as your eyes.)
- Do they have the kind of equipment you want to use? Is the equipment available—or are there long lines and sign-up sheets for popular machines? Are machines in good repair, or do you see many "Out of Order" signs?
- If you'd like to take classes, do they have the ones you want?
- Is the atmosphere right for you? Will you feel comfortable with the other people there? Is the sound level acceptable?
- How long has the facility been in business? Do the professional staff members have the appropriate credentials in their field? (The National Register of Personal Trainers maintains records of qualified and experienced trainers in the UK, they can be contacted on 0181 944 6688.)
- What is the fee? When comparing prices, be sure to include the extras—such as private sessions with a trainer, a permanent locker, towel service, or parking.

how to get this equipment. Maybe you can share with a friend. If you're going to buy dumbbells, find a local store (see page 109). Then make the purchase.

CHOOSE AN AEROBIC ACTIVITY

Though you won't begin aerobic exercise until the third week, start thinking about what you want to do and how you're going to get started. Do you need to buy shoes or workout clothes? A stopwatch? Other equipment? If you're planning to take the walking test, find a measured track.

Are you thinking about joining a gym? If so, have a look at the box on page 210, which will help you select one.

♦ ♦ ♦

I knew I'd like working out on machines, but the idea of joining a gym was intimidating. Would a fat, middle-aged woman feel welcome? It turns out that the real elite at my gym aren't the members with perfect bodies, but the people who show up all the time. One day about a month after I joined, the adorable little fitness instructor who was checking me in—a young woman who was literally half my age and half my size—looked at my attendance record and said, "Wow—you're really happenin' here!"
—Sarah

♦ ♦ ♦

PREPARE FOR THE FOOD PLAN

You'll be exercising just three to six times weekly. But you'll be eating 21 times a week—and more, if you also count snacks. So planning is really important.

Re-read Chapter 9 and decide which food plan to follow in the first week. Come up with ideas for meals: practical breakfasts for weekdays, lunches you can take to the office, dinners your family will enjoy. Think about snacks too: a pick-me-up for your coffee break, something for a long car ride, a quick bite to hold you when you come home hungry and have to prepare dinner. Look at Section IV, which has excellent, practical recipes. A well-stocked pantry will be a big help, so make a shopping list (see box, next page).

SHOPPING LIST

VEGETABLES
- potato
- courgette
- celery
- sweet potato
- onion
- carrot
- mushroom
- broccoli
- cauliflower
- spinach
- green beans
- peas
- aubergine
- cabbage
- lettuce
- green pepper
- cucumber
- tomato
- radish
- spring onions
- dill, parsley
- basil
- other herbs
- garlic
- special in-season vegetables
- canned tomato
- tomato sauce
- vegetable juice

FRUITS AND JUICES
- orange
- grapefruit
- lemon, lime
- apple
- pear
- peach
- plum
- banana
- melon
- pineapple
- mango
- strawberries
- blueberries
- sultanas; dried fruit
- special in-season fruit
- fruit juice

DAIRY
- milk
- yoghurt, low-fat
- cottage cheese, Ricotta
- hard cheese, low fat
- butter
- low-fat sour cream
- sorbet

PROTEINS
- fish, seafood
- chicken, turkey
- steak, mince beef
- eggs
- tofu
- beans—dry, canned

GRAINS
- bread
- pasta
- rice
- couscous
- barley
- oatmeal
- farina
- cereal

OTHER GROCERIES
- dry biscuits, crackers, popcorn
- spices
- balsamic vinegar
- oil, oil spray
- broth
- cocoa powder
- powdered or long-life low-fat milk

OTHER BEVERAGES
- coffee, tea, herbal tea
- mineral water

◆ ◆ ◆

Planning is how I protect myself from those crazy moments when I'm ravenous and standing in front of the open refrigerator, incapable of making sensible decisions about food. The bag of baby carrots is right there. It's like giving myself a willpower transplant.
—Alexandra

◆ ◆ ◆

PLAN YOUR ROUTINE

Now that you've figured out *how*, decide *when*. On which days will you do the strength-training exercises? What about the aerobic activity? Are you going to work out with a friend? If so, make an appointment. What's the best time for you to exercise? Early in the morning? During your lunch break? Before dinner? In the evening?

To the extent possible, create habits and routines for exercise. I realise that a weekly exercise schedule might sound like excessive regimentation, but it's actually very liberating. If you know you're doing strength training while you listen to the morning news every Monday, Wednesday, and Friday, you never have to think about it.

Planning is especially important in the beginning. But it will continue to be helpful, even after you've lost weight. I strongly recommend that you set aside 10 minutes at the start of each week to plan your exercise and meals. You'll be amazed at how much time you save, and how much easier the programme is to follow.

SET UP YOUR LOGS

I've learned from our research projects that record-keeping really helps women follow the programme correctly and remain motivated. Our volunteers agree—even those who weren't convinced at first. In fact, my assistant and I still receive logs from women who finished our studies several years ago.

Make at least ten copies of the exercise and nutrition log forms on pages 215–216 and place them in a folder or notebook. Each form covers a week. I've designed these forms to make record keeping as easy as possible—I'd much rather you spend time exercising than sitting and writing about it.

FOR THE EXERCISE LOGS

On the strength-training log, fill in the dates of each session, and list the weight of the dumbbell or the level for each exercise. Then the next time you won't have a problem remembering all the specifics. Also write down your aerobic exercise: what you did and how many minutes you spent. If you're normally sedentary, you also might want to record your Level 2 activity—remember, the more active you are, the more calories you will burn. (See pages 154–155 for a discussion of aerobic exercise intensity levels.)

FOR THE NUTRITION LOGS

At the beginning of the week, select your food plan—and fill in the top row with the number of portions in each category. (This information is found in the table on page 184.) Then simply make check marks across the row in the relevant box to keep track of what you eat each day. Some women record the portions after each meal; others prefer to fill in the row at the end of the day. I've included space for notes. You might want to jot down a new food or recipe you liked, or keep track of your feelings, or record a special problem or triumph, like successfully managing a holiday dinner. These notes will be very helpful when problems come up and you're trying to devise coping strategies. Later you'll enjoy looking back to reflect on your progress.

TROUBLESHOOTING

Still having difficulty taking that first step? You're not alone. Here are the two start-up issues I hear most often—and my suggestions.

"THIS IS NOT A GOOD TIME FOR ME TO BEGIN A WEIGHT-LOSS PROGRAMME"

Tomorrow night you're having twelve guests for dinner. Or you're about to set off on a two-week holiday. Maybe your dad is in the hospital, and between visits you're scrambling to keep up with your job and kids. So you're absolutely right: this is *not* the best time to start a diet and exercise programme! But let's face it. If you wait for the perfect opportunity—that magic

WEEK _____ Date:_____

Weight (optional): _____

STRENGTH TRAINING LOG			
EXERCISES 2 sets/8 reps	DATE: Pounds or Level	DATE: Pounds or Level	DATE: Pounds or Level
CHAIR STAND			
OVERHEAD PRESS			
BENT-OVER ROW			
CALF RAISE			
SEATED FLY			
ARM CURL			
EXTRA EXERCISES			

AEROBIC EXERCISE LOG		
DAY	ACTIVITY	TIME (minutes)
MONDAY		
TUESDAY		
WEDNESDAY		
THURSDAY		
FRIDAY		
SATURDAY		
SUNDAY		

FOOD LOG

WEEK:	Dairy	Protein	Grain	Fruit	Vegs	Extra	Water
GOALS							8

SUNDAY	Dairy	Protein	Grain	Fruit	Vegs	Extra	Water

Notes:

MONDAY	Dairy	Protein	Grain	Fruit	Vegs	Extra	Water

Notes:

TUESDAY	Dairy	Protein	Grain	Fruit	Vegs	Extra	Water

Notes:

WEDNESDAY	Dairy	Protein	Grain	Fruit	Vegs	Extra	Water

Notes:

THURSDAY	Dairy	Protein	Grain	Fruit	Vegs	Extra	Water

Notes:

FRIDAY	Dairy	Protein	Grain	Fruit	Vegs	Extra	Water

Notes:

SATURDAY	Dairy	Protein	Grain	Fruit	Vegs	Extra	Water

Notes:

moment when you don't have pressure at work, stress at home, holidays or guests—it may never arrive.

Life will always include challenges. If you're going to follow a *lifetime* eating and exercise programme, you'll have to learn how to adapt. So you might as well start now, even if you take just a few steps.

Regina told me:

I'm going on a cruise next week and I want to have fun—I'll go on the programme when I get back.

I wanted Regina to enjoy her cruise. But I knew that over-indulgence could dampen her fun as much as excessive restraint. So I asked her to make five deprivation-free commitments to herself:

♦ Drink at least eight glasses of fluid daily.

♦ Eat at least two portions of fruits and five of vegetables every day—on a cruise, the chef will provide many attractive options.

♦ Set a modest aerobic exercise goal—for instance, to take at least one daily walk around the perimeter of the ship.

♦ Every other day, take five minutes to do the two strengthening exercises that don't require equipment: chair stands and toe stands.

♦ Keep a record—check marks on an index card will suffice—to track success at meeting these goals.

Minor as they might seem, these easy measures will help keep Regina from gaining weight on the cruise. And they'll ease the transition to the full programme once she gets home.

"I CAN'T DO EVERYTHING AT ONCE"

When a woman tells me she feels overwhelmed by the programme, I ask her which of the three components—strength training, aerobic exercise, or the food plan—would be easiest for her to follow. Then I encourage her to work on incorporating that part into her life. Once she does so, she usually finds that she can add the rest.

Dianne had described herself as "a reckless, chaotic eater". Here's how she got started:

> Before I could think about losing weight, I needed to stabilise my eating. This took me a year, and it was an important first step. Then I started strength training. When I had been doing that for a month, I gradually began walking.

HELP—I DON'T HAVE TIME FOR EXERCISE!

When your life is already packed to the limit, fitting in exercise isn't easy. But it's important to your health to find a way. Some possibilities:

- **Exercise while you stay in touch.** Do strength training as you watch (or listen to) the evening TV (or radio) news; use an exercise machine during your favourite TV show. If there's any programme you tune into regularly, make a habit of working out while you watch (or listen).

- **Transport yourself.** Instead of using your car or a bus or a lift, take the opportunity to get some aerobic exercise.

- **Socialise while you work out.** Make exercise dates rather than lunch or dinner dates. This is a great way to spend time with your kids, your companion, your friends—even your parents.

- **Go on the instalment plan.** If you simply can't find 30 consecutive minutes for exercise, divide your workouts into 10-minute segments and squeeze them in when you can. Get up a little earlier in the morning; take a pre-lunch or pre-dinner aerobic break. It all adds up.

For Alexandra, strength training was the key:

I knew I needed to lose weight, and I knew I should be exercising, but I wasn't ready for dieting or aerobics. Strength training appealed to me because it didn't involve sweating or getting down on the floor. After I'd been doing it for a few months, I joined a gym and began aerobic workouts on a treadmill. I wouldn't have felt comfortable joining a gym if I hadn't been strong. Also, around the same time, I began making significant changes in my eating habits. So everything came together eventually.

YOU'RE ON YOUR WAY!

During the first two weeks, you'll begin the food plan and the strength training. Unless you're already doing aerobic exercise (in which case, you should continue), you'll start during Week 3. During the next seven weeks, you'll be settling into the programme. By the tenth week, you'll not only be trimmer, you'll also have new eating and exercise habits that will help you maintain a healthy weight and stay fit for the rest of your life.

If you're accustomed to overly stringent diets and exhausting exercise regimes, you may be sceptical as you begin. How can such a generous food plan and such a light exercise schedule make a difference? Yes, the steps are small at first. But this is a progressive programme, and it will take you as far as you want to go.

STAYING ON TRACK

This is the third time I've lost a lot of weight. The other two times, I felt I had to be perfect, and I was—up to a point. Then everything fell apart completely, and I couldn't pull it back together. This time I haven't been perfect, and oddly enough that's the source of my greatest encouragement. I've seen that I can go on vacation for two weeks—and yes, I skip a couple of workouts and have a few big dinners—but as soon as I get home, I'm right back into my routine. I've returned to the programme after a big party, after a week of house guests, after an illness. So I know that nothing can stop me now.

—Alexandra

◆   ◆   ◆

Have you always found that it's a lot easier to lose weight than to stay slim? This time will be different. You're not going *on* a temporary diet that you'll go *off* the minute you reach a certain weight; you're making permanent changes in your life. New eating and exercise patterns will solidify into habits. Exercise will become a routine part of your day, just like brushing your teeth. You'll reach for the right foods automatically. As this transformation takes place, everything becomes easier and easier.

STAYING POSITIVE

When you begin a new programme, everything seems novel and exciting. Your enthusiasm helps you get started; as you continue, it will keep you going. But this feeling needs to be rekindled from time to time. Let me offer some suggestions.

ENJOY YOUR WORKOUTS

I hope that physical activity becomes one of the great pleasures in your life, as it is in mine. Though my research is about exercise, my workdays at the laboratory are actually very sedentary. Getting outdoors for vigorous activity—hiking, swimming, horseback riding, cycling, running, skiing—makes me feel good. And it's a great way to have fun with my family and friends.

If you find that you're not looking forward to exercising—or that you're even trying to find excuses to skip it—look for a way to refresh your routine. Here are some suggestions:

- **Try new moves**. Have a look at the extra strengthening exercises in Chapter 7 (or in Chapters 8, 11, and 12 of *Strong Women Stay Young*). You might want to change your programme. In Chapter 8, I suggested that you start aerobic exercise with a single "daily bread" activity. But if it becomes a little stale, add variety. If you're walking, try another route, or switch to a bike occasionally. Rent an exercise video one day a fortnight. Changing exercises makes your workouts more interesting, and also helps train different muscles.

- **Recruit a partner.** A workout companion can really help you stick with an exercise programme. Even if you can't find someone who will join you regularly, occasional companionship adds variety to your routine.

- **Create a distraction.** Use a personal stereo to listen to the radio, to recorded music, or to a book on tape. If you're exercising on a machine, you could watch a favourite TV show or a video.

Bon Appetit!

Variety is important for good nutrition, and also for enjoyment. While it's fine to enjoy the same foods every day—such as porridge for breakfast or warm milk at bedtime—don't let yourself get into a rut. If you find you're getting bored with your menus, try these ideas:

- **Plan for variety.** It's easier to expand your repertoire if you have all the necessary foods on hand. Even quick and easy recipes may require thinking ahead. For instance, a baked sweet potato is simple, nutritious, and delicious—but you can't wait until fifteen minutes before dinner to put it in the oven.

- **Shake up your shopping.** Take a little extra time in the grocery store to check out foods you haven't tried before. Find a new kind of whole-grain bread; buy an unfamiliar fruit or vegetable that's in season. Visit a new supermarket or specialty food store. You may discover interesting items in a delicatessen, a bakery, an ethnic grocery or a health-food shop.

- **Look for new recipes.** For starters, check out the terrific menus and recipes in this book. Also try Kreitzman's *Low Fat Cookbook* (Dorling Kindersley)—the recipes are nutritious, practical, and delicious. Another good recipe book is Rosemary Conley's *Low Fat Cookbook* (Century). Magazines are among my favourite sources for new food ideas—check your newsagents or bookshops.

Pain Is a Four-Letter Word

You shouldn't experience acute pain while you're exercising. Nor should you push yourself to a point that leaves you very uncomfortable afterward. Pain isn't going to make your workouts more beneficial—and it certainly won't help you enjoy them. True, you may have a little muscle soreness when you start exercising, especially if you've been sedentary. You'll also feel muscle fatigue at the end of a strength-training set. But any discomfort should be brief. Exercise should make you feel great!

In the Beginning

Your body may need time to adjust to increased activity. During the first few weeks of this programme, or after you return to it following time away, it's normal to feel mild achiness. Discomfort can appear during a workout, or may be delayed until the next day. I don't recommend that you take a painkiller, because medication can interfere with the body's own repair mechanisms. Instead, try hot baths or massage. Stretching can help prevent the problem, and it may also make your sore muscles feel better.

As I'll explain, pain can be a signal that you need medical attention. This doesn't necessarily mean you've been injured by exercising—more likely, you've uncovered an existing problem that was masked by inactivity.

For Strength Training

Learn the difference between "good" pain—which is simply muscle fatigue—and "bad" pain, which can signal an injury. Muscle fatigue is a dull ache that builds up slowly as you lift a weight and vanishes within minutes after you stop. Bad pain is sharp and located in a joint rather than a muscle. It doesn't go away quickly, and feels even worse during your next workout.

If you're experiencing the bad kind of pain while strength training, stop! Relieve the discomfort by elevating the joint and applying ice to it. If pain remains severe, seek medical help. Next time you work out, try lighter weights or a more limited range of motion—whatever it takes to do the exercise comfortably. You can increase slowly from there.

For Aerobic Activity

Strength training will help you minimise discomfort and injuries during aerobic exercise. The same "good pain/bad pain" distinction applies to your aerobic workouts. **If you develop chest pain or tightness, pain down your arm, or severe shortness of breath, stop right away and call your doctor.** These could be symptoms of cardiac problems.

More commonly, women experience pain in their joints—ankles, knees, hips, elbows, or shoulders. Stop any activity that causes sharp pain. Rest the affected area and treat it with ice. In a few days, resume the activity cautiously. See your doctor if the pain persists or gets worse.

SUCCESS ISN'T JUST MEASURED IN KILOS

When you're working toward a goal, self-evaluation helps you succeed. Periodic checks ensure that, if you go off track, you can quickly pull yourself back. Also, your progress is a potent encouragement. Don't just look at the scales: you're making many other positive changes as you create a healthier new lifestyle.

TO WEIGH OR NOT TO WEIGH?

Most health professionals encourage women who are losing weight to step on the scales regularly, but not daily. That's because your weight can vary by one or two kilograms (2 to 4½ lb) in a day because of differences in the amount of water in your body. If you're premenstrual, or if you have eaten salty food and drunk a lot of fluid, you could gain; on a hot summer day, when you're perspiring copiously, you could lose water. These are normal, healthy variations.

In my experience, some women do just fine with daily weighing. They're prepared for variations and can focus on long-term trends. Others avoid the scales and track their progress in other ways. That's okay too. Figure out which approach works best for you.

◆ ◆ ◆

I never get on the scales anymore. If they didn't go down, my con-
fidence would plummet, and that's not good. I look in the mirror;
I go by how my clothes fit. Sometimes my husband will hug me,
notice I feel a little different, and say, "Have you lost weight?"
    –Therese

♦ ♦ ♦

I weigh myself every day, because I have to find out what's going on. I don't overreact to little fluctuations—there could be a lot of reasons for them.
—Nancy

♦ ♦ ♦

One caution if you opt for weekly weigh-ins: don't fall into the trap of crash dieting two days before, and then over-eating right afterwards. The whole point of this programme is to adopt a consistent, healthy eating pattern.

BODY COMPOSITION MEASUREMENTS

Some fitness centres attempt to track weight loss with a tape measure or with devices that claim to gauge body fat, such as infra-red instruments or calipers that measure a fold of skin. Unfortunately, these are usually imprecise. In our laboratory at Tufts, we use more than ten different techniques to measure body composition, including MRIs, CAT scans, and underwater weighing. Believe me, if there were a simple, inexpensive way to do this reliably, we'd use it.

Outside the laboratory, the most accurate way to estimate how much body fat you've lost is to weigh yourself. If you want to try a tape, calipers or another device, wait until you've lost at least 4.5 kilograms (10 lb) before you have yourself re-measured. Otherwise, you may not see a difference.

WATCHING YOUR WORKOUTS

Look for progress in your workouts. With strength training, change is easy to see. During the first ten weeks, the amount of weight you can lift should increase rapidly. Improvements come more slowly after that. But you can flex your biceps muscles and feel your leg muscles—and that's exciting.

You'll also see encouraging changes in your aerobic activity. In just a few weeks you should be able to work out for a longer time without getting tired. You'll probably notice that you have to move faster or otherwise increase the challenge of the activity to reach the correct intensity. That's a sign that your heart and lungs are getting stronger.

Periodically retake the walking test (pages 160–162) to measure improvements in your aerobic fitness. Also review your logs: see where you started and where you are now; compare yourself with the goals on pages 141 (strength training) and page 164 (aerobic activity). Most women are very encouraged by how quickly they progress.

◆ ◆ ◆

The improvement was so dramatic and it happened so fast, I was shocked. Two months after I started strength training, I was using 6.80-kg (15-lb) and 9.00-kg (20-lb) dumbbells. For the first time in years, I could actually see my muscles.
—*Susan*

◆ ◆ ◆

BETTER MEDICAL REPORTS

One of the most satisfying changes that comes with fitness and weight loss is improved health. After your next check-up, compare the latest results with older findings. If your blood pressure, blood cholesterol, and blood sugar were elevated before, they probably will show improvements.

FEELING GOOD

The most important indicator of success is how you feel. Are you less self-critical and happier with yourself? Are you handling stress better? Has your sleep improved? Are you more self-confident? What changes do you see in your everyday life?

◆ ◆ ◆

I have a large garden, and I've just spent three days doing intensive gardening for the first time since I began strength training. This is heavy work, like digging out weeds with a fork. I definitely see a difference. I'm hardly sore; I can easily go up and down the back stairs with a 20-litre (44 pints) watering can. My husband is amazed.
—*Jane*

✦   ✦   ✦

I park on the top floor of the garage at work, on level 6. Now I can run up the stairs without feeling winded—I don't think twice about it. I used to get out of breath at level 4.
—Nancy

✦   ✦   ✦

EVALUATING YOUR PROGRESS

About once a month, use the table below to take inventory. See which pieces of the programme are working well, and which need adjustment.

- **Green light**: You're doing great guns—continue!

- **Yellow light**: You should feel encouraged by the changes you've already made. But you need to do more in order to achieve your goals. Review the relevant chapters to get ideas and new inspiration. You should be in the green light category soon.

- **Red light**: The fact that you did the evaluation is a very good sign, because it means you're ready to get back on track. Do some planning and self-evaluation. What do you want to accomplish? What has worked in the past—and what hasn't worked? What do you need to do now? You may find it helpful to re-read Chapter 5.

DEALING WITH TEMPORARY SETBACKS

It's almost impossible to follow a long-term diet and exercise plan without having problems from time to time. The answer is not to avoid setbacks—that's impossible—but to make sure they're temporary.

How are things going with your –	Green Light	Yellow Light	Flashing Red Light
Strength training	I'm doing the exercises two or three times a week and making progress.	I do the exercises once a week, and I've improved a little.	I haven't been doing the exercises regularly.
Aerobic activity	I'm pretty much following the programme, with three to five workouts a week.	I do at least one workout a week, but don't usually manage as many as three.	I haven't done the workouts for a week or more.
Food plan	I stick to the food plan nearly every day.	I stick to the food plan most of the time.	I haven't really followed the food plan for at least a week.
Weight	I've lost an average of a quarter to a full kilogram (½ to 2 lb) per week.	I've lost a little weight, but not as much as I hoped.	I haven't made progress.
Health and energy	I feel great!	I don't see much difference.	I actually feel worse.

"I CAN'T SEEM TO GET STARTED ON THE EXERCISE PROGRAMME"

One helpful technique is to focus on your motivations. Take the time to write them down. Think about why you want to get fitter and lose weight. Are you trying to look better? Are you concerned about your health because your mother developed diabetes when she was your age? Was your last holiday a disappointment because you didn't have the energy to keep up with your kids? Keep the list of your motivations where you can read it often. You'll be surprised by its power.

♦ ♦ ♦

I had a management job in high tech. The bright 20-year-olds who worked for me looked great, but I felt old and unattractive. It was hard for me to provide leadership, because I didn't feel that I was a desirable person to work for. Losing weight and becoming stronger gave me a whole new identity.
—*Isabel*

♦ ♦ ♦

"I'M DOING A LITTLE EXERCISE, BUT NOT AS MUCH AS I'D LIKE"

Maybe you've started the strength-training programme, but not the aerobics (or the other way round). Or perhaps you're doing both, but less often than you want. I encourage you to continue—you've taken an important first step. Now it's time for the second.

Instead of setting yourself a goal that's a little too difficult, then feeling guilty when you fail, come up with an objective so easy that you're certain of success. Let's say you've been meaning to start strength training, but weeks have gone by and it just hasn't happened. Stop expecting to begin the entire programme straight away—that expectation isn't working. Instead, promise yourself that this week you'll do the two exercises that don't require equipment, the chair stands and the toe raises. Then, next week, continue those exercises and buy the dumbbells. If you go that far, I bet you'll be doing the entire programme a week or two later. There's nothing as motivating as setting a goal and achieving it.

"I'VE STARTED THE FOOD PLAN A COUPLE OF TIMES, BUT I CAN'T STICK WITH IT"

Starting and stopping is discouraging. It's better to follow a few aspects of the programme consistently, even if you can't manage the whole thing. For instance, resolve to drink at least eight glasses of water a day, or promise yourself to switch to whole-grain breads and cereals. Just concentrate on the changes you find possible. Once those are in place, other pieces of the programme will seem much easier.

"EVERYTHING WAS GOING BEAUTIFULLY— THEN I WENT ON HOLIDAYS"

Brief interruptions won't keep you from your goal, provided you learn to recover quickly. Since interruptions are an unavoidable part of life, this is an important skill for permanent weight loss. And now you have the perfect opportunity to practise. The key is to get back on track as soon as you can— and to feel really good about that.

Dianne, one of the women who tested the programme for this book, sounded very disheartened at one of our Monday meetings. She told the group, "I was at a barbecue over the weekend, and I really blew it." Someone asked her, "Exactly what did you eat?" As Dianne recited the list, she began to realise that she hadn't done as badly as she'd thought. Yes, she'd eaten too much chicken, too much cake, and too much in general—but she'd skipped the chips and taken a modest portion of potato salad. She had eaten much less than she would have a year ago. And even more important, she'd returned to her food plan the very next day. As I reminded her, "One meal is inconsequential when you think of your life as a whole."

◆ ◆ ◆

When I travel, I enjoy checking out other gyms. This usually costs between five and ten pounds per visit. It's fun to go to a posh fitness centre with a friend, and visit on side-by-side treadmills instead of at the dinner table.
—Sarah

◆ ◆ ◆

THE HUNGER CHECKLIST

Hunger is not only normal—it's desirable. Your body is reminding you to eat. You should feel hungry when you wake up in the morning and haven't eaten since the day before; you should feel hungry three to five hours after a meal. Unfortunately, hunger is an imperfect mechanism. It's not immediately relieved by eating, and sometimes it's confused with other feelings.

Use this hunger checklist to decode the urge to eat:

♦ **When did I last eat?** If your last meal was less than three hours ago, you probably don't need to eat again. Also, remember that it takes your body at least 20 minutes to "register" a meal; if you've just eaten, allow yourself enough time to feel full.

♦ **Have I had enough to drink?** Sometimes what feels like hunger is really thirst. You should be drinking at least eight glasses of fluid a day. If you feel hungry less than three hours after a meal, try drinking a glass of water.

♦ **Am I tired?** If you're fatigued, you may be looking for a quick pick-me-up. Try a nap instead of a snack—you'll be surprised at how refreshing a brief rest can be. If fatigue is a frequent problem, adjust your schedule so you get enough sleep.

♦ **Am I under stress?** When you're anxious or upset, eating can be a form of comfort and self-sedation. Instead, try a walk or some other exercise to cope. And make an effort to identify the underlying source of your distress.

As you lose weight, you'll learn to identify real hunger and distinguish it from these impostors. Gradually your desire for food will become more attuned to your body's true needs.

"I'M DOING EVERYTHING RIGHT, BUT I HAVEN'T LOST ANY WEIGHT!"

If you're following the programme consistently, you'd think that your weight loss would be consistent too, but that's not always the case. It's perfectly normal to lose weight for a few weeks, level off for a few weeks, then start losing again. We're not sure why this happens. Some women retain water and gain weight just before their periods, then lose it afterwards; they learn to expect this pattern.

Try not to be discouraged—you're doing something very positive for yourself, and probably just need to give it a little more time. Meanwhile, consider whether either of these factors might account for the disappointing results:

Am I eating more than I realise?

This is usually the problem when people tell me they're following the food plan but not losing weight. Don't drop down to a lower calorie level until you check portion sizes. Take a look at page 195 (the portion primer).

Food	Recorded as	But Actually	Extra Calories (approximate)
Porridge for breakfast	200 g (7 oz)	300 g (11 oz)	60
Whole meal bread for sandwich at lunch—two thick slices cut from a bakery loaf	60 g (2 oz) (2 30-g slices)	125 g (4 oz) (each slice was about 60 g)	120
Chicken breast	85 g (3 oz)	120 g (4 oz)	40
Apple	1 medium	1 large	30
Dry biscuits with low-fat cheese spread (free sample at shop)	Not recorded	½ Grain ½ Dairy	80
Broken biscuit pieces (nibbled as she set out biscuits in a bowl)	Not recorded	¼ Grain	20

Lillian lost 4.5 kilograms (10 lb) in the first 12 weeks, then hit a plateau. "I'm following the programme religiously!" she told me—and she was. She was doing the exercises perfectly, and her food diary showed the right number of portions every day. I asked her to try weighing and measuring for a few days, just in case.

Next week Lillian was back—three-quarters of a kilo (1½ lb) lighter. She'd checked her portions with scales and measuring cups, and had been startled to discover that she was eating more than she intended. As she listed the discrepancies, I tallied the extra calories. She hadn't counted them—but her body certainly had.

A series of minor slips—see table on previous page—added up to an extra 350 calories in a single day! As soon as Lillian trimmed portion size and included all snacks as part of her meal plan, her weight loss resumed. If this hadn't happened, I would have suggested that she switch to the next lower food plan—1200 calories instead of 1600.

Am I exercising at sufficient intensity?

If you are, you should be making progress. With strength training, that means graduating to heavier weights during the first few months (progress normally slows after that). With aerobics, you should be able to increase the distance, intensity, or length of your workouts, especially in the early months.

If you are not seeing changes, you might need to push yourself a little more—provided you can do so comfortably. Your aerobic workouts should raise a sweat. If they don't, check your pulse and review the exercise intensity scale (page 155).

What if you can't find an explanation? If you're following the 1200 calories plan and doing the exercises but are not losing weight, give yourself a couple of weeks. If you're still at a plateau, talk to your doctor. Medications and medical problems can cause weight gain or explain why you are not losing weight on a sensible diet-plus-exercise programme.

◆ ◆ ◆

I was on a 1200-calorie diet, and gaining weight. First two pounds the next week another pound. The third week, when the scales were up a pound yet again, I went to my doctor. "I'm not surprised," she told me. "You're pregnant."
—Alexandra

◆ ◆ ◆

"MY FRIENDS FEEL GREAT ON THIS PROGRAMME, BUT I'M DRAGGING"

You're wise to be concerned. Try to figure out what's going on. You might have to adjust the programme—or the problem could lie elsewhere.

◆ **Are you eating enough?** If you're losing more than a kilogram (2 lb) a week, or if you're losing less but feel hungry all the time, you may need more food. Just move up to the next higher calorie level. If you're already at 2000 calories, add more foods from the Next-to-Nothing list (page 192). Also check portions to be sure you are not giving yourself too little.

◆ **Are you drinking enough?** You need at least eight glasses of fluid a day—and more during the summer when it's hot.

◆ **Are you exercising too much?** Proper training should make you feel energised, not exhausted, at the end of the day. If your muscles continue to feel sore, stiff, or fatigued after the first few weeks, you may be pushing too hard. Experiment with a lighter schedule to see if that restores your energy—cut back on either the intensity or duration of exercise. Don't forget to take off one day per week.

IF YOU WERE PREVIOUSLY ON A VERY LOW-CALORIE DIET . . .

Your metabolic system went into starvation mode, which is nature's way of helping you survive when your food supply is inadequate. Now your body will need several weeks to re-adjust. In the meantime, you may not lose weight—indeed, you might even gain a kilogram or two (2 to 4½ lb). Try to be patient. Once you start eating well and exercising, your metabolism should get back up to speed, and your weight loss should resume. Even before that, you should see other benefits: more energy and strength, less stress, better sleep. Focus on these improvements, which show that you're doing something good for yourself.

- **Do you have a mild illness?** Give yourself a week to feel better. If you haven't improved by then, see your doctor. Sometimes a cold or other malady can sap your energy, even though it's not bad enough to send you to bed. Another possibility is that increased physical activity has uncovered a condition you didn't notice before, such as borderline anaemia.

- **Are you under stress?** Look at what else is going on in your life. Pressures at work or at home could be affecting your energy.

AFTER THE FIRST TEN WEEKS

No matter how much weight you need to lose, the end of the tenth week is an important milestone. Take some time to think about—and enjoy—what you've accomplished: you've lost weight, you've established healthy eating habits, you've become stronger and fitter. These are wonderful gifts to yourself.

To Continue Losing Weight

If you've been losing a quarter to a full kilogram (2 lb) a week, just keep doing what you're doing. If your weight loss has slowed to less than a quarter kilogram (1/2 lb) per week but you're close to your goal, I suggest you continue your programme and be content to progress more slowly.

Sometimes weight loss stalls when you're still far from finished. Check portion size. If that's not the answer, you'll need to decrease your calorie intake, increase your aerobic exercise, or do a little of both.

To Decrease Intake

Drop to the next lower calorie plan. You don't have to take the entire step at once. For example, if you're on the 1600-calorie plan, you can go to 1200-calorie during the week but continue eating 1600 calories on the weekends. If you're following the 1200-calorie plan already, don't go any lower. Either increase your exercise or try to adjust your expectations so that you're satisfied with slower change.

To Increase Exercise

Add Level 3 aerobic activity—but don't exceed one hour daily. Continue to take at least one day a week off to give your body a rest. Make sure you're getting plenty of Level 2 aerobic activity. The more you can do, the better.

If you want to add extra strengthening exercises, use the ones in this book or from *Strong Women Stay Young*. Don't work the same muscles two days in a row; they need time to rest and repair themselves.

Adjust Your Goals

Sometimes weight loss stops when you're still heavier than you want to be. You try cutting back on food, but skimpier rations leave you hungry. Adding aerobic exercise isn't appealing either—you're already working out five days a week, for a total of five hours. This situation calls for re-assessment of your weight loss goals.

If the issue is appearance rather than health, perhaps you should decide to be content at your present weight. There are many other ways to improve how you look—consider what you might accomplish with different clothing, a haircut, new glasses, or makeup. What if you've reached a weight that puts you at risk according to the BMI chart? Maintain your good eating and exercise habits, but try to increase your Level 2 aerobic activity: cultivate

The Last 2 Kilograms

When you're just 2 kilograms (4½ lb) from your goal and nothing is happening, it's easy to feel impatient. Don't be tempted to take drastic measures—they rarely work in the long run. Continue following the programme, but drop down to the next lower calorie level and increase physical activity.

What if the weight still doesn't budge? Ask yourself if you've *ever* been able to maintain a lower weight than you're at right now. If not, maybe your body is trying to tell you something. Try this: decide to live with your present weight for a month or two. Just concentrate on eating well and exercising. A kilo (2 lb) or so extra may slip away. Or you might find that you're content with your new shape. With more muscle and less fat, your body will look slimmer than you might expect at a given weight.

an active hobby; walk more often during the day. The extra calories you burn will contribute to continuing slow weight loss.

WHEN YOU'VE REACHED THE WEIGHT YOU WANT TO MAINTAIN

I hope you're proud of yourself, because you deserve to be. You've lost weight— and lost it the right way, through healthy, positive change. For many women, this achievement signals that they can take on other challenging tasks.

What you've learned so far will be of enormous help. But there are three new areas to think about:

FINE-TUNING THE PROGRAMME

To maintain your weight, you'll have to adjust your programme. Here are things to consider as you add and subtract:

Strength Training

Some women enjoy strength training so much, they're not only eager to continue with three sessions per week but even want to add new exercises. That's just fine. However, when you're maintaining your weight, two sessions a week is sufficient.

Aerobic Exercise

You can continue your present exercise programme, or cut back a little. But to stay fit, do at least 20 minutes of Level 3 aerobic activity three days a week. The more you exercise—and that includes Level 2 activity—the more you'll be able to eat without regaining.

Food Plan

If you want to continue exercising at your present level, you'll have to eat more to maintain your weight. Move to the next higher calorie level and see how that works. You can make the change gradually. Remain at your present level during the week and increase it only on weekends.

Listening to Your Appetite

During the weeks—or maybe months or years—of weight loss, you've eaten slightly less than your body needs. This has required you to tame your natural appetite. Now your appetite must perform its natural task, which is to regulate your food intake so that it matches your energy expenditure. If you've been overweight for a long time, you may not trust your appetite at first. Focus on learning what hunger feels like, and how quickly your body registers satiation. With continuing success, you'll gain confidence.

◆　◆　◆

I'm making healthier choices just because that's what I prefer now. I went out for a buffet dinner on my birthday, and it wasn't a struggle to skip the creamy seafood sauce. I felt very good about that.
—Ruth

◆　◆　◆

Safeguarding Your Success

Once you reach the weight you'd like to maintain, I suggest you weigh yourself periodically. It's all too easy for the grams to creep back; this can happen slowly. Since you might not notice a change in your clothing immediately, the scales provide the best early warning.

Don't avoid weighing yourself because you're afraid you'll see a number you won't like. It's much better to confront the problem straightaway. And it's important to check, regardless of what else is happening in your life. The time you're most likely to gain is during change and disruption—when you switch jobs, begin or end a relationship, give birth, become ill, or take a holiday.

Everyone slips now and then. Don't be self-critical if that happens. Focus on all the positive things you've been able to accomplish. If you could do all this, you can certainly get back on track.

QUESTIONS AND
ANSWERS

You have to figure out ways to stay motivated. Since that can change, you need to take time to focus on yourself and think about what you're doing. It's easy to slip back into old routines. I find it helpful to re-read things that have been motivating—that gives me a little shot in the arm.

—Dianne

◆ ◆ ◆

As I wrote this book, I tried hard to anticipate your concerns. I hope that if any questions remain, they're answered here. Also, check the index in case you missed a detail. After you've been following the programme for a few months, I suggest you glance over the book again. As you lose weight and gain experience with the exercise and food plans, different information will become relevant.

IF YOU HAVE QUESTIONS ABOUT THE *STRONG WOMEN STAY SLIM* PROGRAMME

Q: I have a medical condition—can I still do this programme?

A: Nearly everyone can do this programme, even people who have recently had surgery—including hysterectomy, mastectomy, and other cancer treatment—as well as those with chronic but *stable* medical conditions, such as heart disease, diabetes, arthritis, osteoporosis and joint problems. If you have a specific health concern, here are my recommendations:

- Each individual is unique. It's *very* important to discuss the programme with your doctor before you start, so you can make any necessary adjustments in the food or exercise plan.

- Start conservatively and progress slowly. For instance, if you have problem shoulders, you can begin by doing the strengthening exercises without dumbbells; if that's comfortable, you can try 1.35-kg (3-lb) dumbbells, increasing the weights every two weeks instead of weekly.

- Pay attention to your body. Feeling good is your best indicator that you're exercising properly.

Q: I've just had a baby and I'm eager to get back to my pre-pregnancy weight. When can I start this programme?

A: At your postpartum check-up—usually four to six weeks after birth—talk to your doctor about starting this programme and losing weight. If you're healthy and doing well, you'll probably get an okay. Of course, you'll need to modify the food plan if you're breastfeeding, because you need extra calories and calcium. Start slowly and progress conservatively, because you're probably more out of shape than you expect. Even before your check-up, you can begin making healthy changes in your life. As soon as you feel able, take walks with your new baby. Eat plenty of vegetables, and drink at least eight glasses of fluid per day.

Q: I look fine if I'm sitting down, but I desperately need to do something about my hips. Can this programme help?

A: Many people ask me how to focus weight loss on a particular part of the body. I wish it were possible! Strength training can firm specific muscles, and that makes a big difference. But it can't selectively eliminate the fat covering the muscles. The only way to get rid of fat (short of surgery) is to lose weight, and you can't target that.

The chair stands (see page 116) will tighten your buttocks and give you slimmer hips. Whole-body aerobic activity, such as walking, preferentially decreases abdominal fat, which is the type most detrimental for health; weight loss will help too. Remember that basic body shape seems to be part of our genetic heritage. Once you've reached a healthy weight and have accomplished what's possible with strength training and aerobic exercise, I hope you'll learn to love your feminine curves.

Q: Will this programme eliminate my upper arm "bat wings"?

A: Strengthening exercise will tone and strengthen your arm muscles; aerobic exercise will decrease the fat layer on top of them. Many women are delighted by these changes; they tell me that their upper arms look better than they have in decades. By losing weight slowly, you give the skin of your upper arms more time to tighten up.

Q: Can my husband do this programme with me?

A: Definitely! The food plan, which is based on the Food Guide Pyramid, is designed to help everyone eat well. Men, like women, are advised to get at least 30 minutes of aerobic exercise a day. If your husband is currently sedentary, he can use the instructions in this book to work up gradually to that. Many men—including my husband—do the strength-training exercises and gain a lot of benefit from them. Because of their greater muscle mass, most men are able to start strength training with heavier weights, and they usually reach a higher level than women do. But the basic instructions are the same: how to make the moves, the number of sets and reps and the number of sessions per week, what intensity of effort to aim for, and how to progress.

FOR YOUR DOCTOR

Here are some of the studies and articles that underlie the *Strong Women Stay Slim* programme.

◆ Miriam E. Nelson *et al.*, "Effects of high-intensity strength training on multiple risk factors for osteoporotic fractures: a randomized controlled trial", *Journal of the American Medical Association* 1994, volume 272, pages 1909–14.

◆ Douglas L. Ballor and Eric T. Poehlman, "Exercise-training enhances fat-free mass preservation during diet-induced weight loss: a meta analytical finding", *International Journal of Obesity* 1994, volume 18, number 1, pages 35–40.

◆ Ross E. Andersen *et al.*, "Encouraging patients to become more physically active: the physician's role", *Annals of Internal Medicine* 1997, volume 127, pages 395–400.

◆ Steven N. Blair *et al.*, "Influences of cardiorespiratory fitness and other precursors on cardiovascular disease and all-cause mortality in men and women", *Journal of the American Medical Association* 1996, volume 273, number 3, pages 205–10.

◆ Wayne W. Campbell *et al.*, "Increased energy requirements and changes in body composition with resistance training in older adults", *American Journal of Clinical Nutrition* 1994, volume 60, pages 167–75.

◆ Mary L. Clem *et al.*, "A descriptive study of individuals successful at long-term maintenance of substantial weight loss", *American Journal of Clinical Nutrition* 1997, volume 66, pages 239–46.

IF YOU HAVE QUESTIONS ABOUT YOUR WEIGHT

Q: Every time I try to lose weight, I get derailed by hunger. I'm thinking about trying an appetite suppressant. What would you suggest?

A: When women ask me about appetite suppressants, I urge them to try other measures first—drinking more fluids, eating more high-fibre foods (fruit, vegetables, and whole grains), and doing aerobic exercise. Eating well and being physically active really help curb the appetite, and they have so many other positive effects. It's not clear that appetite suppressants really help in the long run—if they do, you might need to continue taking them for the rest of your life and there's always a risk of unexpected side effects. This is just as true of herbal substitutes as it is for conventional drugs.

Prozac and other anti-depressants are sometimes prescribed for weight loss because they affect serotonin levels in the brain. These are very powerful drugs, and should be taken only after careful discussion with a well-informed doctor.

Q: I'm bloated, so I look fatter than I am—help!

A: Some women retain water and feel uncomfortably bloated. This can happen before your period or when you're going through menopause. Here are a few suggestions:

- ◆ Cut back on salt. Most of us don't need to limit salt, but we typically eat far more than our body needs. Cutting back can't hurt, and it might help. Limit or eliminate high-salt condiments, such as pickles. Leave the salt shaker off the table—try a dash of lemon juice or a sprinkle of pepper or herbs instead.

- ◆ Do aerobic exercise. Physical activity improves the body's water regulation.

- ◆ Don't restrict fluids. When intake is reduced, your body will reduce output to match.

Q: I read an article that said it's important not to get heavier as I get older. But then I saw another article that said it's healthy to gain with age. Which is right?

A: This is a matter of continuing controversy. Some studies show that gaining ½ to 1 kilogram (1 to 2 lb) per decade is beneficial because it reduces the risk of developing osteoporosis and becoming frail. But other studies find that the healthiest people are those who maintain the same body weight throughout their lives. Everyone agrees, however, that gaining more than 5 to 10 kilograms (11 to 22 lb) as you get older puts you at greater risk for heart disease, stroke, diabetes, osteoarthritis, and other conditions.

Q: Every year I begin to gain weight in autumn, then lose most of it in the spring. What's going on?

A: This is a common pattern, and there are several possible explanations. During the colder and darker months of the year, we tend to spend more time indoors and become less active. At the same time we may eat a little more, especially during the holiday season. Some people are more prone to depression during the winter, which further contributes to both inactivity and increased eating. Fortunately, these changes are usually reversed in the spring, as we become more active. You can counter winter weight gain (and depression) by remaining physically active throughout the year.

IF YOU HAVE QUESTIONS ABOUT STRENGTH TRAINING OR AEROBIC EXERCISE

Q: Won't I get bulky if I lift weights?

A: No—you'll gain a lot of strength, but your muscles will be only slightly larger. When you combine strength training with aerobic exercise and weight loss, you shed body fat. Since a kilo of fat takes up more space than a kilo of muscle, even women who don't lose weight often drop a dress size or two.

HOW I ENCOURAGE MY CHILDREN TO BE PHYSICALLY ACTIVE

My husband and I love sport, and we're fortunate that our three children—ages 6, 8 and 9—share this great pleasure. Much of what we do together as a family involves getting outdoors for vigorous physical activity.

At the weekends we head for Vermont and New Hampshire, where our parents live—ideal spots for family hikes. Last summer my husband and I, our two oldest children, and my brother-in-law and his two teenage daughters took a challenging twelve-kilometre (7½ miles) climb in the White Mountains. What a wonderful day! At the top, we enjoyed a spectacular view and feasted on wild blueberries. Our reward at the end was a swim in a magnificent emerald pool at the bottom of the mountain.

In the summer, when we're not hiking, we're usually in the water. When my son was 7, he did a kilometre-long (½ mile) swim with me along the edge of a New Hampshire lake. In the winter, we switch to skiing, both downhill and cross-country. And when the local pond freezes over, we go ice-skating.

Since our kids love the water, we joined a local indoor pool so they can swim year-round. In the evenings when I jog, my son accompanies me on his bike and we have a great time. Sometimes we run silly races in the backyard, laughing as we go around certain trees and keeping track of our time just for fun. Now that the children are getting older, the whole family is beginning to play tennis—I think it's especially important to encourage youngsters to play sports that can last a lifetime. On rainy days, my husband and I push the living-room furniture to the walls and bring out a long jump-rope. All the kids in the neighbourhood love jumping rope in our living room!

Q: This book suggests two sets of eight reps for strength training—but another book I have recommends twelve reps. What's best?

A: Most experts agree that the best way to improve strength is with two or three sets of six to twelve repetitions. But no one knows just what the optimal mix of sets and reps is. I know from our research that two sets of eight reps can increase strength and build muscle and bone. Women find that this workout is practical and uses their time efficiently, which is important too.

Q: Will I perform better if I eat health bars and drink athletic beverages?

A: These foods and drinks may help elite athletes get through tough endurance events like triathlons. But there's no evidence that they're better than ordinary drinks or food for the health and performance of the average active woman.

Q: Can my children do these exercises?

A: Aerobic and strengthening activities are great for kids, but paediatricians do not recommend that children use free weights or exercise machines. That's because youngsters are more prone to injury than adults, and also are more likely to misuse equipment. Encourage your children to walk, run, use a skipping rope, dance, swim, and play sport. To build strength, they can do the toe stands and chair stands from this book, which don't use equipment. Other appropriate strengthening exercises are sit-ups, push-ups, pull-ups, stationary jumps, and hill runs. Most important of all is to have fun, so that your kids gain a lifelong love of physical activity.

IF YOU HAVE QUESTIONS ABOUT THE FOOD PLAN

Q: I like to have a late dinner, but I've read that this interferes with weight loss. Is that true?

A: Many nutritionists speculate that this is true, based on experience with their clients—but it hasn't yet been confirmed by research. In any case, it's generally a good idea to have your last meal at least two hours before you go to bed. This enables you to digest most of your food before you become horizontal. Your gastrointestinal system works best when you're upright, because gravity helps move things along. You may have noticed that you're more likely to get heartburn if you lie down soon after a meal. Or you might have had the experience of going to bed after a big dinner, and the next morning you have the uncomfortable feeling that the meal hasn't moved very far. For these reasons it's best not to eat a heavy meal just before you go to bed.

Q: I'm a nurse, and I'm on different shifts throughout the month. Any suggestions?

A: You definitely face an extra challenge. Planning becomes even more important when your schedule changes so much. If you don't think ahead, you may be stuck with fast food because you're hungry in the middle of the night and that's all you can find.

To help yourself get organised, come up with a workable meal schedule for each shift. Try not to have your main meal too close to bedtime. Also, work out when to shop. Develop a repertoire of wholesome packed specialties: sandwiches with wholegrain bread; soups and stews that can be warmed in the microwave, if you have access to one; crispy salads; ready-to-eat fruit. Don't neglect fluids. Keep supplies of appealing drinks on hand, like herbal teas and flavoured mineral water.

Q: I weigh more than 136 kilos (300 lb), and even 8400 kilojoules leave me hungry. Can I eat more and still lose weight?

A: Perhaps. But first make sure you're eating as much satisfying food as the 2000 calories plan allows. Select whole grains, which are high in satiating fibre. Choose tofu and fish for your protein, so you can enjoy larger portions. Take full advantage of the Next-to-Nothing list (pages 192–194), which allows very generous quantities of filling vegetables that don't add many calories. If all this still leaves you hungry, try supplementing your daily plan with two fruits or a fruit and a vegetable.

Q: Can I use a sugar substitute?

A: You can, but I don't recommend it. First, there's not much evidence that sugar substitutes help with long-term weight control. Adding a substitute to coffee instead of sugar saves you just 12 calories, not a significant amount. Second, there are nagging questions about safety and side effects. But most important: when you use substitutes, you are not allowing yourself to develop the healthier food preferences that will make it much easier to stay slim. Women who cut back on sugar without resorting to substitutes may feel deprived at first. But after a brief period, they almost always find that their cravings for sweet foods diminish.

Q: Sometimes I have to eat at a fast-food restaurant. Can you give me any recommendations?

A: Check the menu carefully. Order fruits and salad or vegetables if possible, and select the leanest option for your main dish. Have a large glass of water or a calorie-free drink. Servings may be large—take that into account when you figure out your portions for the day. If you find you're often eating at fast food restaurants where it's hard to follow your food plan, take some time to figure out alternatives. Maybe you can bring food from home or find other restaurants. If it's just an occasional meal, simply do your best to adapt and don't worry about it.

Q: I know I should eat three well-balanced meals, but some days I just don't have time. Is it okay to eat a meal replacement bar instead of breakfast or lunch?

A: In the long run, it's best for you to organise your day and week so you can eat real food. An occasional replacement won't do any harm—and it's certainly better than grabbing a chocolate bar. However, whole foods bring so much more to your diet; they're healthier and more satisfying.

Q: I don't always want all my Extras—but I'd like additional fruit or meat. Is there any way to substitute?

A: Yes. Instead of using the Extras for fats, sweets, or alcohol, you may exchange them for additional portions of the other food groups, as follows:

1 Dairy portion	=	2 Extras
1 Protein portion	=	1 Extra
1 Grain portion	=	2 Extras
2 Vegetable portions	=	1 Extra
1 Fruit portion	=	2 Extras

Q: I don't eat meat. Can I substitute dairy foods for proteins?

A: It's fine to substitute 1 Dairy for 2 Proteins, because dairy foods contain high-quality protein. However, since the foods in the Protein list aren't high in calcium, you can't swap in the other direction.

Q: I love potatoes—but if I eat a big potato, I use up my Vegetable portions and that doesn't seem like a good idea.

A: You're right—you need other vegetables too. What you can do is to substitute two portions of potato for a Grain. For example, a small potato, which is two Vegetable portions, can be counted as one Grain.

Q: My kids and husband won't eat this food, so I'm making different meals for everyone. It's like running a restaurant—what can I do?

A: As a mother, I can really sympathise. Fortunately, this is a very flexible food plan, so you should be able to make it work for everyone. It's also a healthy way of eating that will benefit other members of your family. Here are a few suggestions:

- Find a compromise between convenience and individual preferences. I serve one meal for dinner, but my husband and kids can have their own choices at other meals.

- Get your children (and husband) involved in meal planning and cooking.

- Encourage your kids to try new foods.

- Have very simple foods on hand—cereals, fruits, bread—when you're serving something that one family member dislikes.

Q: I'm lactose intolerant—how can I get enough calcium?

A: Dairy products contain a sugar called lactose that some people can't easily digest. Lactose intolerance could be the problem if you develop gas, cramps or other gastrointestinal problems after consuming dairy foods. These suggestions might help:

- Have just half a portion of dairy food at a time. You may be able to tolerate small quantities without distress.

- Buy products to which lactase has been added—that's the enzyme that digests lactose. Or buy the enzyme, which comes in pill form (available in pharmacies and health food shops), and consume it along with dairy portions.

- Select dairy foods that don't contain undigested lactose, such as cheese or yoghurt made with live cultures.

- If the above suggestions don't work, get calcium from non-dairy sources, such as calcium-fortified orange juice or soy milk, tofu made with calcium sulphate, canned fish with bones, collard greens, broccoli, or spinach.

Q: I want to take a calcium supplement—which kind is best?

A: The two best types are calcium carbonate and calcium citrate. Select either, but calcium carbonate supplements should be taken with a meal, since the stomach acid released during digestion helps with absorption.

"I LIKE VEGETABLES, BUT I FIND IT HARD TO EAT THE RECOMMENDED AMOUNT"

It's a common problem. Most of us enjoy eating vegetables a lot more than we enjoy preparing them. Here are some tips from women who've followed this food plan:

- Use raw veggies for snacks, like baby carrots or broccoli florets.
- Eat vegetables in the form of soups and juice. One-portion cans of vegetable juice make great snacks for the car or office.
- Buy bagged, ready-to-eat lettuce to streamline salad preparation.
- Use supermarket vegetables, not only for salads but also for snacks, stir-fries, and cooked side dishes.
- Learn how to prepare vegetables quickly in the microwave.
- Try having vegetables at breakfast. For instance, add chopped vegetables to an omelette.
- Grate vegetables into soups, casseroles, meat loaf, homemade breads, and even cakes.

HOW TO COPE WITH BUFFETS AND BANQUETS

Delicious food is an important part of celebrations, holidays and other special occasions. But temptation can be a problem. Here are some suggestions from women in the group that tested this programme:

- Provide low-calorie options. If you're the hostess, make extra salads or vegetable side dishes. If you're a guest, offer to bring a fruit salad for dessert or a low-fat dip and veggies for an appetiser.
- Fill up with a bowl of vegetable soup or a salad half an hour before the party.
- Eat very, very slowly.
- Delay helping yourself at a buffet; postpone taking second helpings. You'll probably eat less because you have less time—also, the food may run out.
- Cruise a buffet table before filling your plate, and take only the items you really want.
- Forget the "clean plate club"—don't eat anything you don't really enjoy.
- At a cocktail party or buffet, stand with your back to the food and talk a lot!
- Send extras home with your guests, or ask a friend to help you put them away quickly. Clean-up is often the most difficult time if you're the hostess, because it's hard to resist leftovers when you're no longer distracted by the party.

TROUBLESHOOTING

Q: I went to a brunch buffet and ate much more than I intended. What should I do about dinner?

A: The fact that you're ready to resume your food plan means that the brunch will have no long-term consequences. Don't skip dinner—that could lead to excessive hunger and more problems the next day. Just eat lightly.

Q: My friend and I started the programme together five weeks ago. She's lost 4.5 kilos (10 lb) but I've only lost 1.5 (3½ lb), and I'm getting very discouraged.

A: Please don't be unhappy—you've lost 1.5 kilograms (3½ lb), which is terrific! You have to realise that everyone is different. If your friend is much younger or much heavier than you are, her resting metabolic rate is almost certainly higher. There may be subtle differences in her food choices, or she may be burning extra calories because she does more Level 2 activity. Try to focus on your own excellent progress: you've lost weight, and you're gaining important benefits by eating better and exercising. Stick with it, and you'll continue to lose weight.

Q: I've just recovered from the flu. How soon can I resume my workouts?

A: Don't try to lose weight while you're sick. Stop exercising and take care of yourself. Once you're over the illness—when you no longer have a fever or feel sick—start back slowly. Cut the intensity and time of your workouts in half, and see how that goes. If you feel fine, work back up to your previous level. That could take just a week or two if you had a cold, or longer if your illness was more severe.

Q: I was doing well—then I had a family crisis and stopped exercising for two months. I want to get going again, but I'm not sure where to start.

A: Your earlier success will be a great help. You already have the dumbbells; you know the strength training moves; you've selected an aerobic activity. However, you can't expect to resume at the same point you reached before. Reduce the intensity of your exercise sessions: with strength training, drop down a level or use a weight that's half of what you were lifting before. With aerobic activity, decrease the time by half (but don't do less than 10 minutes). You'll quickly bounce back. In two or three weeks you'll be where you were before, and ready to progress.

FOR MORE INFORMATION

There are many very good resources for people interested in weight loss, nutrition, and exercise. If you want to learn more about how strength training affects muscles, bones, and balance, you might want to read my first book, *Strong Women Stay Young* (Aurum Press, 1997).

Excellent books on nutrition are:

◆ *The Tufts University guide to Total Nutrition,* by Stanley Gershoff, Ph.D, with Catherine Whitney (Harper perennial, 1990)

◆ *Food Facts & Figures: A Comprehensive Guide to Healthy Eating,* by Jill Davies and John Dickerson (Faber & Faber, 1989)

◆ *ABC of Nutrition,* Edited by A. S. Truswell (BMJ Publishing Group, 1992)

◆ *The Right Way to Eat,* by Miriam Polunin (J. M. Dent, 1978)

The following two sports nutrition books are written for athletes and active adults:

◆ *The Complete Guide to Sports Nutrition,* by Anita Bean (A & C Black, 1993).

◆ *Foods, Nutrition and Sports Performance,* (Journal of Sports Sciences, 1991)

IV

MENUS AND RECIPES
BY STEVEN RAICHLEN

INTRODUCTION BY MIRIAM NELSON

I love to eat good food. In the summer, I enjoy luscious ripe fruit and crispy vegetables (especially the sweet carrots that my kids pull from my brother-in-law's garden); in the winter I savour hearty soup and just-baked whole-grain bread. Special dinners with family and friends are high points in my life. I'm always looking for new recipes that are wholesome but also delicious. Some of my favourites come from Steven Raichlen, author of the *High-Flavor, Low-Fat* cookbooks. He has a special knack for creating dishes that delight the tastebuds while trimming excess calories. So when I decided to include menus and recipes in this book, I turned to Steven.

I requested exciting, enticing recipes but reminded him that most of us can't spend hours in the kitchen. I wanted to expand my repertoire—I confess that I sometimes fall into a rut and wind up making the same few dishes over and over. However, I'm slightly intimidated by long lists of exotic ingredients. I asked for suggestions that could introduce variety, such as unusual fruits and vegetables, flavourful teas and interesting spices, but without a lot of effort.

Steven was intrigued by the challenge of working within the food plan. He came up with ten remarkable menus that contain just 1200 calories for an entire day of flavour-packed eating (plus simple additions for those on the 1600- or 2000-calorie plans). I hope you'll be thrilled to see how well you can eat on the *Strong Women* programme. This is the kind of food I'd expect at a world-class health resort!

If you were a resort chef, you might follow these ten menus over the next couple of weeks, but we really don't expect you to do that. If you're like me, when you make a big casserole over the weekend, you want to coast on the leftovers during the week. And since I don't have unlimited pantry space, I tend to buy just one or two types of tea and use those up before I get another. But I hope you'll return again and again to these menus—and to the individual recipes—when you want to add zest to your meals. They're an inspiration.

This chapter proves that healthy can be delectable and that you don't have to give up wonderful food to lose weight. Bon appétit!

In case you're wondering . . .

- **About snacks:** All the daily menus include meals plus snacks. Sometimes there's just one snack, sometimes there are several—and the time of day varies too. Feel free to adapt the day's allotment to your preferences. For example, you could move a morning snack to afternoon, or add an evening snack by saving dessert from lunch or dinner.

- **About beverages:** If a beverage isn't specified for a meal or snack, have a glass of water or another Next-to-Nothing drink. Remember, it's important to get enough fluids, both for health and for satiety.

- **About portions:** For menu items that are made from recipes, eat one serving and count portions as the recipe indicates. For other items, such as mashed potatoes or low-fat yoghurt, eat one portion (see Chapter 9 for portion sizes) unless otherwise indicated.

- **About exotic ingredients:** A large supermarket should have just about all the items called for in these menus and recipes. You could also try a health food or a gourmet food shop for unusual spices, cereals, teas, fruits, types of rice, and frozen wholegrain waffles.

A Vegetarian Feast

BREAKFAST

Cream of wheat cereal with blueberry syrup (page 308)
Indian spice tea

LUNCH

Mexican bean salad with pumpkin seeds (page 279)
Tortilla crisps (page 275)
Fruit juice spritzer (page 304)

SNACK

1 orange

DINNER

Green salad with balsamic vinegar
Garlic bread
Spaghetti primavera with grilled vegetables (page 287)
Sliced mango

For the 1600 plan: Add 150 g (5 oz) diced melon to breakfast; add 7 crackers to morning snack; add 2 tablespoons hummus and celery sticks to afternoon snack; double portion of Spaghetti Primavera.

For the 2000 plan: Add 150 g (5 oz) diced melon to breakfast; add 7 crackers to morning snack; double serving of Tortilla Crisps; add 2 tablespoons hummus and celery sticks to afternoon snack; double portion of Spaghetti Primavera; double portion of Garlic Bread; double portion of salad; add evening snack of 1 tablespoon peanut butter on sliced Granny Smith apple.

Quick and Easy

BREAKFAST
Fruit juice spritzer (page 304)
Muesli parfait (page 308)

SNACK
Tamari popcorn (page 275)
Lemon mineral water

LUNCH
Tomato juice
Carrot sticks
Roast beef sandwich (page 284)

DINNER
Spicy ginger turkey stir-fry (page 294)
Brown rice
Melon salad with yoghurt and mint (page 298)
Iced green tea

SNACK
Chocolate milk
Cinnamon crackers

For the 1200 plan: Have 200 g (7 oz) brown rice at dinner.

For the 1600 plan: Add extra 30 g (1 oz) roast beef to sandwich; add nectarine to lunch; add afternoon snack of 3 tablespoons salsa, 30 g (1 oz) Tortilla Crisps (page 275), 30 g (1 oz) low-fat Cheddar.

For the 2000 plan: Add extra 60 g (2 oz) roast beef and 1 slice of bread to sandwich; add nectarine to lunch; add afternoon snack of 6 tablespoons salsa, 60 g (2 oz) Tortilla Crisps (page 275), 30 g (1 oz) Cheddar; double Melon Salad portion for dinner.

Delectably Different

———————— ⌢ ————————

BREAKFAST

Orange juice
Mexican scrambled egg with toasted tortillas (page 306)
Café de olla (page 305)

LUNCH

Mushroom and goat's cheese sandwich (page 285)
Iced tea with fresh mint

SNACK

Low-fat chocolate yoghurt

DINNER

Bulgur salad with tomato and mint (page 277)
Fish en papillote (page 297)
Pear

———————— ⌢ ————————

For the 1600 plan: Double portion of scrambled egg at breakfast; at lunch, increase goat's cheese to 60 g (2 oz) and add 150 g (5 oz) sliced strawberries.

For the 2000 plan: Double portion of scrambled egg at breakfast; add mid-morning snack of 1 tablespoon peanut butter with celery sticks and sliced apple; at lunch, increase goat's cheese to 60g (2 oz) and add 150 g (5 oz) sliced strawberries and a small handful of nuts; add a wholemeal roll to dinner; add evening snack of hot chocolate.

A Summer Sizzler

BREAKFAST

Peach yoghurt smoothie (page 304)
Multigrain toast

SNACK

Carrot and celery sticks

LUNCH

Gazpacho salad (page 280)
Garlic pitta chips (page 276)
Next-to-nothing mushroom pâté (page 273)
Iced raspberry tea

SNACK

Low-fat strawberry yoghurt

DINNER

Moroccan lamb kebabs (page 293)
Lemon couscous (page 283)
Blueberry soup (page 300)
Mint tea

For the 1600 plan: Add a sliced apple to morning snack; increase Gazpacho Salad to 500 ml (1 pint) at lunch and add 50 g (2 oz) vanilla pudding; increase lamb to 150 g (5 oz) at dinner.

For the 2000 plan: Add extra slice of bread and 2 tablespoons low-fat cream cheese to breakfast; add sliced apple to veggie stick snack and double the vegetable serving; increase Gazpacho Salad to 250 ml (½ pint) at lunch and add 50 g (2 oz) vanilla pudding; increase lamb to 150 g (5 oz) at dinner; add evening snack of 3 tablespoons peanuts, 2 tablespoons raisins, and 30 g (1 oz) pretzels.

A Weekend Celebration

BREAKFAST

Wholegrain waffles
Apple sauce
Café latte (page 306)

LUNCH

Vegetable sticks
Hungarian cheese dip (page 274)
Vegetable juice

DINNER

Garlic soup (page 276)
Paella Valenciana (page 288)
Peaches in sparkling wine (page 303)

For the 1600 plan: To lunch, add sandwich of 30 g (1 oz) pitta, 2 tablespoons hummus, with diced lettuce, tomato, and green pepper; add afternoon snack of lemon yoghurt with 75 g (3 oz) diced fruit.

For the 8400 plan: Add extra waffles and 50 g (2 oz) apple sauce to breakfast; to lunch, add sandwich of 60 g (2 oz) pitta, 4 tablespoons of hummus, with diced lettuce, tomato, and green pepper; add afternoon snack of lemon yoghurt with 75 g (3 oz) diced fruit; add 2 plain biscuits at dinner.

East Meets West

BREAKFAST

Shredded wheat cereal with skimmed milk
Sliced pear
Apple spice tea

LUNCH

Chicken broth
Pitta chips (page 276) with Asian bean dip (page 272)

SNACK

Flavoured fruit yoghurt

DINNER

Marinated mushroom kebabs (page 272)
Shabu-shabu with lemon-ginger dipping sauce (page 295)
Jasmine rice
Strawberry napoleons (page 301)

For the 1200 plan: Have 200 g (7 oz) jasmine rice at dinner.

For the 1600 plan: Add mid-morning snack of 60 g (2 oz) low-fat cottage cheese and 75 g (3 oz) pineapple chunks; at lunch, increase Bean Dip to 150 g (5 oz) and Pitta Chips to 2 portions, and add carrot sticks; add crackers to afternoon snack.

For the 2000 plan: Add 60 g (2 oz) bagel, 2 tablespoons of low-fat cream cheese, and 2 teaspoons of jam to breakfast; add mid-morning snack of 60 g (2 oz) low-fat cottage cheese and 75 g (3 oz) pineapple chunks; at lunch, increase Bean Dip to 1 cup and Pitta Chips to 2 portions, and add carrot sticks and 1 small nectarine; add crackers to afternoon snack; at dinner, double the portion of mushrooms and increase protein to 120g (4 oz).

Something Exotic

BREAKFAST
*Puffed rice cereal with milk and sliced fresh fruit
Vietnamese iced coffee (page 305)*

SNACK
*Slice of wholemeal cinnamon raisin bread
Mineral water*

LUNCH
*Bulgur lettuce roll-up with spicy yoghurt dipping sauce
(page 278)
Iced ginseng tea*

SNACK
Indian milk shake (page 303)

DINNER
*Teriyaki salmon with spicy slaw (page 290)
Boiled rice
Coconut fruit salad (page 300)*

For the 1200 plan: Have 200 g (7 oz) boiled rice at dinner.

For the 1600 plan: Add a slice of raisin bread to morning snack; add fresh orange and 125 ml (¼ pint) yoghurt to lunch; for dinner, increase salmon to 150g (5 oz) and slaw to 200g (7 oz).

For the 2000 plan: Add a slice of raisin bread to morning snack; add fresh orange and 125 ml (¼ pint) yoghurt to lunch; add dinner appetiser of 4 celery stalks stuffed with 2 tablespoons low-fat cream cheese, and increase salmon to 185g (6 oz) and slaw to 200 g (7 oz); add evening snack of wholemeal English muffin with 2 teaspoons of honey and a banana.

Winter Warmer

BREAKFAST

Porridge with brown sugar
Apple
English breakfast tea

LUNCH

Veggie melt (page 285)
Sparkling mineral water with lemon

SNACK

1 slice raisin bread with low-fat cream cheese

DINNER

Sliced cucumber sprinkled with fresh dill
Paprika chicken (page 286)
Poppy seed pasta (page 283)
Nectarine orange

LATE NIGHT COMFORT

Hot chocolate

For the 1600 plan: Increase breakfast porridge to 200 g (7 oz) made with 250 ml (½ pint) skimmed milk and 2 teaspoons of brown sugar; add 1 pear to lunch; increase dinner chicken serving by 30 g (1 oz).

For the 2000 plan: Increase breakfast porridge to 200 g (7 oz) made with 250 ml (½ pint) skimmed milk and 2 teaspoons of brown sugar; add 1 apple and a second slice of bread and cream cheese portion to mid-morning snack; add 1 pear to lunch; increase chicken serving by 60 g (2 oz) and double portions of pasta and vegetables at dinner.

Vegetarian Favourites

BREAKFAST

Muesli with chopped apple
Earl Grey tea

LUNCH

Greek salad sandwich (page 284)
Iced mint tea with lemon

SNACK

Low-fat yoghurt

DINNER

San Antonio slaw (page 281)
Three-bean chilli (page 289)
Polenta
Nectarine or other fruit in season

For the 1600 plan: Add mid-morning snack of 30 g (1 oz) Spiced Walnuts (page 275); at lunch, add second Greek salad sandwich and a navel orange.

For the 2000 plan: Add mid-morning snack of 60g (2 oz) Spiced Walnuts (page 275); at lunch, add second Greek salad sandwich and an orange; add sliced banana to afternoon yoghurt snack; at dinner, double polenta to 125 g (4 oz) and add 100 g (4 oz) of slaw.

A Mediterranean Celebration

BREAKFAST

Grapefruit half
Cinnamon-orange popover with jam (page 307)
English breakfast tea

LUNCH

Fusilli salad with cherry tomatoes and rocket (page 282)
Ryvitas
Tangerine with low-fat yoghurt

SNACK

Broccoli
Garlic-yoghurt dip (page 274)

DINNER

Mixed salad with balsamic vinegar
Bouillabaisse with garlic toasts (page 292)
Orange custard (page 299)
Espresso

For the 1600 plan: Add 2 teaspoons jam for breakfast; for mid-morning snack, add sandwich made with 1 slice wholemeal bread, 30 g (1 oz) turkey, 30 g (1 oz) cheese, and 1 sliced apple; for dinner, increase salad serving to 200 g (7 oz).

For the 2000 plan: Add 1 popover and 2 teaspoons jam for breakfast; for mid-morning snack, add sandwich made with 2 slices wholemeal bread, 30 g (1 oz) turkey, 30 g (1 oz) cheese, and 1 sliced apple; double broccoli in afternoon snack; increase salad serving to 200 g (7 oz) for dinner; add evening snack of 7 crackers and 50 g (2 oz) dried fruit.

APPETISERS AND SNACKS

SALADS AND SIDE DISHES

SANDWICHES

ENTRÉES

DESSERTS

BEVERAGES

BREAKFASTS

Asian Bean Dip

The Far East meets the Middle East in this Asian twist on hummus. Serve the dip with vegetable chips, rice crackers or toasted pitta chips. Hoisin sauce, a Chinese condiment made with soybeans, is available at most super-markets.

> 1 400g (14 oz) can chickpeas, drained, rinsed with cold water and drained again
> 1 garlic clove, minced
> 2 spring onions, finely chopped
> 2 teaspoons grated fresh ginger
> $1^1/_2$ tablespoons soy sauce
> 1 tablespoon hoisin sauce (if unavailable, use 2 teaspoons more soy sauce and $^1/_2$ teaspoon more sugar)
> 1 tablespoon rice vinegar or distilled white vinegar
> 2 teaspoons sugar

Combine the ingredients in a food processor and purée until smooth. Season to taste, adding soy sauce or sugar as needed.

Makes four 100 g (4 oz) servings

PER SERVING: 1 PROTEIN

Marinated Mushroom Kebabs

Mushrooms make a great Next-to-Nothing snack. This recipe is modelled on the French hors d'oeuvre *champignons à la Grecque* (in the style of Greece).

> 400g (14 oz) mushrooms (choose small mushrooms that are all the same size)
> 8 pearl onions, cut in half
> 175 ml ($^1/_3$ pint) dry white wine
> 175 ml ($^1/_3$ pint) vegetable or defatted chicken stock
> 3 tablespoons fresh lemon juice

1 tablespoon tomato paste
2 teaspoons ground coriander
$^1/_2$ teaspoon black pepper
1 bay leaf
Salt to taste

1. Wipe the mushrooms clean with a damp cloth and trim off the ends of the stems. In a deep saucepan, bring the onions, wine, chicken stock, lemon juice, tomato paste, coriander, pepper, and bay leaf to a boil.
2. Add the mushrooms and briskly simmer until the mushrooms and onions are tender and the cooking liquid is slightly reduced, about 15 minutes, stirring often. Add salt—and more lemon juice if needed—to taste. Transfer the mushrooms and liquid to a bowl and cool to room temperature, then refrigerate until cold.
3. Serve the mushrooms and onions with bamboo skewers for picking them up. Or, if you like, thread the mushrooms and onions on bamboo skewers to make kebabs.

Makes four servings

Per serving: 1 Vegetable or Next-to-Nothing

Next-to-Nothing Mushroom Pâté

Here's a mushroom spread that's loaded with flavour, not fat. The secret is to roast the vegetables in a hot oven to concentrate their flavour.

250g (9 oz) button mushrooms, trimmed and quartered
$^1/_2$ small onion, peeled and quartered
2 garlic cloves, peeled
1 teaspoon olive oil
Salt and freshly ground black pepper
2 tablespoons finely chopped parsley (preferably Italian)
2 teaspoons cognac (optional)
1–2 tablespoons dried breadcrumbs, or as needed

1. Preheat the oven to 230°C (450°F). Place the mushrooms, onion and

garlic in a non-stick roasting pan. Toss with the olive oil, salt and pepper. Roast the mushrooms until nicely browned, 15–20 minutes, stirring to ensure even cooking. Let the mushrooms cool to room temperature.

2. Purée the vegetables in a food processor, adding the parsley, cognac and salt and pepper to taste. If the spread seems too wet, add a tablespoon or two of breadcrumbs.

Makes eight 30g (1 oz) servings

PER SERVING: NEXT-TO-NOTHING OR 1 VEGETABLE

Garlic-Yoghurt Dip

60 ml (2¹/₂ fl oz) low-fat plain yoghurt
1 garlic clove, crushed
¹/₄ teaspoon grated lemon zest
Salt and freshly ground pepper

Combine the yoghurt, garlic and lemon zest. Add salt and pepper to taste.

Makes one 60 ml (2¹/₂ fl oz) serving

PER SERVING: ¹/₄ DAIRY

Hungarian Cheese Dip

250g (9 oz) low-fat cottage cheese
¹/₂ teaspoon onion powder
¹/₂ teaspoon garlic powder
¹/₂ teaspoon paprika
¹/₂ teaspoon dry mustard
Salt and freshly ground pepper to taste

Purée cottage cheese in a food processor with the onion powder, garlic powder, paprika, and dry mustard. Add salt and pepper to taste.

Makes two 150 g (5 oz) servings

PER SERVING: 1 DAIRY

Spiced Walnuts

> 3 tablespoons walnuts
> Olive oil cooking spray
> A pinch of garlic salt
> A pinch of pepper
> A pinch of paprika
> A pinch of cumin

Spray the walnuts with olive oil. Toss with the garlic salt, pepper, paprika, and cumin.

Makes one serving

PER SERVING: 1 PROTEIN, 1 EXTRA

Tamari Popcorn

Tamari is a naturally brewed soy sauce available in health food or Asian food shops.

> 75 g (3 oz) natural-flavoured popcorn
> 3 tablespoons tamari

Sprinkle the popcorn with the tamari.

Makes one serving

PER SERVING: 1 GRAIN

Tortilla Crisps

> 1 flour tortilla
> A pinch of chilli powder
> A pinch of garlic salt

Cut a flour tortilla into wedges and sprinkle with chilli powder and garlic salt. Bake on a non-stick baking sheet in a preheated 200°C (400°F) oven until crisp, 3–5 minutes.

Makes one serving

PER SERVING: 1 GRAIN

Garlic Bread

> 1 2¹/₂ cm (1 inch) thick slice of French bread
> Olive oil cooking spray
> 1 minced garlic clove or ¹/₄ teaspoon garlic powder
> 1 teaspoon Parmesan cheese

Spray the bread with olive oil and sprinkle with the minced garlic (or garlic powder) and Parmesan. Preheat the oven to 175°C (350°F) and bake for about 10 minutes, or until crisp and golden brown, turning once.

Makes one serving

PER SERVING: 1 GRAIN

Garlic Pitta Chips

> 30 g (1 oz) pitta bread
> ¹/₄ teaspoon garlic powder or garlic salt

Open the pitta bread to form 2 rounds. Cut into wedges and sprinkle with the garlic powder or garlic salt. Preheat an oven to 200°C (400°F) and bake until crisp, about 5–8 minutes.

Makes one serving

PER SERVING: 1 GRAIN

Garlic Soup

Garlic Soup is a Castilian speciality—and a reputed remedy for a hangover. Don't be alarmed by the amount of garlic, a whole head. Cooking greatly reduces its pungency. To make a vegetarian garlic soup, simply omit the ham and use vegetable stock.

> 4 teaspoons olive oil
> 1 head garlic, broken into cloves, peeled, and thinly sliced

30 g (1 oz) lean prosciutto or lean bacon, cut into matchstick slivers
   (optional)
1 tablespoon Spanish paprika
1 litre (2 pints) defatted chicken or vegetable stock
Salt and freshly ground black pepper
4 2¹/₂ cm (1 inch) thick slices French bread
2 tablespoons chopped Italian parsley

1. Heat olive oil in a large non-stick saucepan. Add the garlic and cook over medium heat until lightly browned, about 2 minutes. Stir in the prosciutto or bacon and paprika and cook for 1 minute. Add the stock and bring to a boil. Simmer the soup until richly flavoured, about 5 minutes. Add salt and pepper to taste.

2. Meanwhile darkly toast the bread in a toaster or under the grill. (Darkly toasting gives the bread a smoky flavour, which makes the soup taste richer, too.)

3. To serve, place a slice of bread in each of the four soup bowls. (The soup would be served in an earthenware bowl in Spain.) Ladle the soup on top, sprinkle with parsley, and serve.

Makes four 250 ml (¹/₂ pint) servings

PER SERVING: 1 GRAIN, 1 EXTRA

Bulgur Salad with Tomato and Mint

Bulgur (cracked wheat) is a versatile grain, ideal for summer dishes. You don't even have to turn on the stove to cook it: simply soak it in cold water until tender. This takes about 8 hours. Start with soaking the bulgur before you go to work so it will be ready when you come home for dinner. Then the salad can be assembled in a matter of minutes.

Note: This recipe calls for more salad than you'll need for dinner. The extra can be used in a Bulgur Lettuce Roll-Up (page 278), which you can prepare for lunch the following day.

350 g (12 oz) bulgur
2 cucumbers, seeded and diced

2 ripe tomatoes, seeded and diced

4 sprigs finely chopped Italian parsley

3 sprigs chopped fresh mint or 1 tablespoon dried mint

4 spring onions, finely chopped

1 garlic clove, minced

60 (2$^1\!/_2$ fl oz) ml fresh lemon juice

$^1\!/_2$ teaspoon ground cumin

Salt and freshly ground black pepper

4 lettuce leaves, for serving

4 sprigs of Italian parsley (garnish)

1. Rinse the bulgur in a strainer and transfer to a large bowl. Add 1 litre (2 pints) cold water. Let soak in the refrigerator until tender and tripled in bulk, 6–8 hours.

2. Drain the bulgur in a strainer, pressing with the back of a spoon to extract the excess water. Combine the bulgur, cucumber, tomatoes, parsley, mint, spring onions, garlic, lemon juice and cumin in a mixing bowl and toss to mix. Add salt, pepper, and cumin to taste. (At this point you may like to set 100 g (4 oz) of salad aside for Bulgur Lettuce Roll-up.)

3. To serve, place a lettuce leaf on each of 4 salad plates. Mound the bulgur salad in the centre and garnish each serving with a sprig of parsley.

Makes four 375 g (13 oz) dinner servings and one 250 ml (9 oz) lunch serving

PER LUNCH SERVING: 1 GRAIN, 1 VEGETABLE

PER DINNER SERVING: 2 GRAINS, 1 VEGETABLE

Bulgur Lettuce Roll-Up with Spicy Yoghurt Dipping Sauce

I like to think of this quick, easy lunch as a Middle-Eastern burrito. The filling is left-over bulgur salad.

For the roll-up

3 large lettuce leaves (cos or iceberg)

150 g (5 oz) Bulgur Salad (page 277)

1 carrot, thinly sliced lengthwise
1 stalk celery, thinly sliced lengthwise
$1/2$ red pepper, thinly sliced
1 spring onion, green tops only
$1/2$ tomato, cut into wedges

For the Yoghurt Dipping Sauce
125 ml ($1/4$ pint) plain low-fat yoghurt
$1/2$ garlic clove, minced
$1/4$ teaspoon grated lemon zest
$1/4$ teaspoon ground cumin
$1/4$ teaspoon hot paprika or cayenne
Salt and freshly ground black pepper

1. To make the roll-up, lay the lettuce leaves on a cutting board, one slightly overlapping the other. Spread the bulgur salad in the centre. Lay the carrot, celery, pepper, spring onion, and tomato on top, running lengthwise. Starting at one side, roll the lettuce into a compact roll.
2. To make the dipping sauce, whisk together the yoghurt, garlic, lemon zest, cumin, and paprika in a small bowl, adding salt and pepper to taste. Use the sauce as a dip for the lettuce roll as you eat it.

Makes one serving

PER SERVING: 1 GRAIN, 2 VEGETABLE, $1/2$ DAIRY

Mexican Bean Salad with Pumpkin Seeds

This salad is bursting with colours and flavours. It's simple too, and I think you'll find the combination of kidney beans and pumpkin seeds delicious.

1 kg (2 lb) cooked pinto or kidney beans
    (if canned, rinse well to remove excess salt)
60g (2 oz) toasted pumpkin seeds
1 yellow pepper, diced
1 cucumber, seeded and diced

½ red onion, diced
1–2 jalapeño chillies, finely chopped
  (for a milder salad, seed the chillies)
3 tablespoons chopped fresh coriander
2 tablespoons red wine vinegar
1 tablespoon lime juice
4 teaspoons olive oil
2 teaspoons brown sugar
Salt and freshly ground black pepper

Drain the beans in a colander, rinse well, and drain again. Combine beans and the other ingredients in a bowl and toss to mix. Adjust the seasoning, adding lime juice or salt to taste.

Makes four 300 g (10 oz) servings

Per serving: 3 Proteins, 1 Vegetable, 2 Extras

Gazpacho Salad

Gazpacho is the world's most famous chilled soup. The unique combination of vegetables thickened with diced bread set me thinking about a salad that could be made with these ingredients.

2 tablespoons red wine vinegar
3 tablespoons defatted chicken or vegetable stock
4 teaspoons extra-virgin olive oil
Salt and freshly ground black pepper

1 cucumber, peeled, seeded, and cut into 1 cm (½ inch) dice
2 juicy ripe tomatoes, cut into 1 cm (½ inch) dice
1 green pepper, cut into 1 cm (½ inch) dice
2 stalks celery, cut into 1 cm (½ inch) pieces
½ red onion, finely chopped
1–2 garlic cloves, minced
4 slices country-style bread, cut into 1 cm (½ inch) cubes

1. In a salad bowl, whisk together the vinegar, stock and oil. Add salt and pepper to taste.

2. Stir in the cucumber, tomatoes, pepper, celery, onion, garlic, and bread. Let the salad stand for 10 minutes. Adjust the seasoning, adding salt or vinegar to taste.

Makes four 150 g (5 oz) to 200 g (7 oz) servings

PER SERVING: 1 GRAIN, 1 VEGETABLE, 1 EXTRA

San Antonio Slaw

200g (7 oz) shredded green cabbage
2 small horseradishes, cut into matchstick strips
$^1/_2$ large peach or mango, cut into matchstick strips
1 green chilli or $^1/_2$ green pepper, cut into thin strips
1 carrot, cut into matchstick strips
3 sprigs chopped fresh coriander
3 tablespoons diced red onion
1–4 fresh or pickled jalapeño chillies, thinly sliced (the hotter, the better!)
1 garlic clove, minced
3 tablespoons fresh lime juice, or to taste
1 tablespoon honey
Salt and freshly ground black pepper

Combine all the ingredients in a mixing bowl and toss to mix. Adjust the seasoning, adding salt, sugar or lime juice to taste.

Makes four 250 g (9 oz) servings

PER SERVING: 1 VEGETABLE OR NEXT-TO-NOTHING

Fusilli Salad with Cherry Tomatoes and Rocket

Rocket (arugula) gives this pasta salad a distinctive peppery bite. Fusilli are coiled or spring-shaped pasta.

> 250 g (9 oz) dried fusilli
> Salt
> 1 1/2 tablespoons balsamic vinegar
> 1 1/2 tablespoons defatted chicken or vegetable stock
> 4 teaspoons extra-virgin olive oil
> 1 garlic clove, minced
> Freshly ground black pepper
> 300 g (11 oz) ripe cherry tomatoes, halved
> 1 large bunch rocket, washed, dried, and cut crosswise into 1 cm
>   (1/2 inch) strips
> 1 tablespoon capers, drained
> 1/2 teaspoon hot chilli flakes

1. Cook the fusilli in plenty of rapidly boiling salted water until *al dente*, about 8 minutes. Drain the pasta in a colander, refresh under cold water, and drain well again.
2. In an attractive salad bowl, whisk together the vinegar, stock, oil, garlic, and salt and pepper to taste. (Whisk until the salt dissolves.) Add the pasta, tomatoes, rocket, capers, and chilli flakes and toss to mix. Adjust the seasoning, adding salt or vinegar to taste. The pasta should be highly seasoned.

Makes four 250 g (9 oz) servings

PER SERVING: 2 GRAINS, 1 VEGETABLE, 1 EXTRA

Lemon Couscous

Couscous looks like a grain but actually it's a type of semolina. This North African staple is very easy to prepare. You can find couscous in the grain or pasta section of any supermarket.

> 1 garlic clove, minced
> 1 shallot or $1/2$ small onion, minced
> 1 teaspoon grated lemon zest
> 2 tablespoons chopped parsley
> 625 ml ($1^{1}/4$ pints) vegetable or defatted chicken stock
> 475 g (1 lb) dry couscous
> Salt and freshly ground pepper

1. In a large frying pan combine the garlic, shallot or onion, lemon zest, parsley and stock and gently simmer for 5 minutes.
2. Remove the pan from the heat and stir in the couscous, salt and pepper. Cover the pan and let stand for 10 minutes, or until the couscous is soft. Fluff the couscous with a fork before serving, adding salt and pepper to taste.

Makes four 250 g (9 oz) servings

PER SERVING: 2 GRAINS

Poppy Seed Pasta

> 250 g (9 oz) cooked pasta of your choice
> 60 ml ($2^{1}/2$ fl oz) low-fat sour cream
> 2 teaspoons poppy seeds

Toss the noodles with the sour cream and poppy seeds.

Makes four 250 g (9 oz) servings

PER SERVING: 2 GRAINS

Roast Beef Sandwich

      1 slice of wholegrain bread
      $1/2$ teaspoon wholegrain mustard
      $1/2$ teaspoon prepared horseradish
      3 lettuce leaves
      30g (1 oz) lean roast beef
      3 tomato slices
      100 g (4 oz) radish or alfalfa sprouts

Generously spread a slice of wholegrain bread with mustard and horse-radish. Place the lettuce leaves and roast beef on top. Top the sandwich with the tomato slices and sprouts.

Makes one serving

PER SERVING: 1 GRAIN, 1 PROTEIN

Greek Salad Sandwich

      30 g (1 oz) pitta bread
      Cos lettuce
      Tomato slices
      Sliced red onion
      Chopped spring onions
      Fresh dill sprigs
      1 tablespoon lemon juice
      30 g (1 oz) feta cheese

Stuff a pitta bread with cos lettuce, tomato, red onion, spring onions, and dill. Sprinkle with lemon juice and crumbled feta cheese.

Makes one serving

PER SERVING: 1 GRAIN, 1 VEGETABLE, 1 DAIRY, 1 EXTRA

Veggie Melt

1 slice of pumpernickel bread
Wholegrain mustard
3 tomato slices
3 apple slices
30 g (1 oz) Cheddar cheese
Freshly ground black pepper

Spread a slice of pumpernickel with wholegrain mustard. Top with the tomato and apple. Place cheese on top and sprinkle with freshly ground black pepper. Cook under a grill or in a toaster oven until the cheese melts.

Makes one serving

PER SERVING: 1 GRAIN, 1 DAIRY

Mushroom and Goat's Cheese Sandwich

4 mushrooms, preferably with medium-sized caps
1 garlic clove, cut into matchstick strips
Salt and pepper
1 multigrain roll
30g (1 oz) goat's cheese, softened
$1/2$ bunch watercress
3 tomato slices

Stud the mushroom caps with garlic and season with salt and pepper. Grill the mushrooms until nicely browned and tender, about 4 minutes per side. Cut the roll in half, spread with goat's cheese, and fill with the mushroom, watercress, and tomato slices.

Makes one serving

PER SERVING: 2 GRAINS, 1 DAIRY, 1 EXTRA

Paprika Chicken

Here's a low-fat remake of a Hungarian classic. For the best results, use Hungarian paprika, which is available at gourmet shops and many super-markets.

> 500g (1 lb) skinless, boneless chicken breasts,
>   thinly sliced across the grain
> Salt and freshly ground black pepper
> 1 tablespoon sweet paprika or to taste
> 2 teaspoons olive oil
> 1 onion, finely chopped
> 2 garlic cloves, finely chopped
> 1 red pepper, finely chopped
> 1 tomato, finely chopped
> 1 tablespoon flour
> 250 ml (½ pint) defatted chicken stock
> 250 ml (½ pint) low-fat sour cream
> 2 tablespoons chopped Italian parsley (garnish, optional)

1. Place the chicken in a bowl and season with salt, pepper, and half the paprika. Toss to mix. Let stand for 5 minutes.
2. Meanwhile, heat the oil in a large non-stick frying pan. Add the onion, garlic, and pepper and cook over medium heat until the vegetables are soft and just beginning to brown, about 5 minutes, stirring often. Add the tomatoes after 3 minutes. Stir in the flour and remaining paprika and cook for 1 minute.
3. Stir in the chicken and cook for 1 minute. Stir in the stock and most of the sour cream, reserving 2 tablespoons for garnish. Gently simmer until the chicken is cooked and the sauce is nicely thickened, 8–10 minutes. Add more salt, pepper and paprika as needed to taste.
4. Transfer the chicken to plates or a platter. Garnish with dollops of sour cream and sprinkle with parsley.

Makes four servings

PER SERVING: 4 PROTEINS, 1 VEGETABLE, 1 EXTRA

Spaghetti Primavera with Grilled Vegetables

One of the best ways to create big, mouth-watering flavours with a mini-mum of fat is to use cooking methods that add flavour, like grilling. These grilled vegetables give this pasta so much flavour, you won't miss the heavy cream in the original. The sauce is made by simmering stock and low-fat sour cream.

Grilled Vegetables

    1 courgette, cut diagonally into thick slices
    1 yellow squash, cut diagonally into thick slices
    1 onion, cut into thick slices
    Olive oil spray (or a paper towel dipped in 1 teaspoon olive oil)
    Salt and freshly ground black pepper

    125g (4 oz) spaghetti

Sauce

    4 teaspoons extra-virgin olive oil
    2 shallots or small onion, finely chopped
    2 garlic cloves, finely chopped
    1 tomato, seeded and finely chopped
    250 ml ($^{1}/_{2}$ pint) defatted chicken or vegetable stock
    250 ml ($^{1}/_{2}$ pint) low-fat sour cream
    8 fresh basil leaves, thinly sliced
    Freshly ground black pepper
    A pinch of cayenne pepper
    90 g (3 oz) freshly grated Parmesan
    4 whole basil leaves (garnish)

1. Preheat the barbecue grill or broiler. Spray the courgette, squash, and onion slices with oil (or wipe them with an oiled paper towel). Season with salt and pepper to taste. Grill the courgette, squash, and onion slices until nicely browned on both sides, 3 to 4 minutes per side. Transfer to a platter.

2. Cook the pasta in plenty of lightly salted boiling water until *al dente*, 8 minutes.

3. Meanwhile, heat the olive oil in a non-stick frying pan. Cook the shallots or onion and garlic until fragrant but not brown, about 2 minutes. Add the tomato and cook for 1 minute. Thinly slice the grilled vegetables, add them to the pan, and cook for 1 minute.

4. Add the chicken stock and sour cream. Boil briskly for 5 to 8 minutes, or until well reduced, thickened and richly flavoured. Stir in the basil and pasta and cook until thoroughly heated, 2 minutes, turning with tongs. Adjust the seasoning, adding salt and pepper to taste.

5. Spoon the pasta into bowls and sprinkle with the cheese and basil.

Makes four servings

Per serving: 1 Grain, 1 Dairy, 1 Vegetable, 1 Extra

Paella Valenciana

Paella is a colourful Spanish rice dish that is ideal for entertaining. You will need a short, starchy grain like the Italian arborio rice for this.

> 1 tablespoon extra-virgin olive oil
> 1 onion, finely chopped
> 2 garlic cloves, minced
> ¹/₂ red pepper, cut into ¹/₂ cm (¹/₄ inch) strips
> ¹/₂ yellow pepper, cut into ¹/₂ cm (¹/₄ inch) strips
> 1 ripe tomato, seeded and cut into ¹/₂ cm (¹/₄ inch) dice
> 185g (6 oz) boneless, skinless chicken breasts, cut into
>   2¹/₂ cm (1 inch) pieces
> 400 g (14 oz) arborio rice
> 125 ml (¹/₄ pint) dry white wine
> 1 litre (2 pints) defatted chicken stock or vegetable stock, or as needed
> ¹/₂ teaspoon saffron threads, soaked in 1 tablespoon hot water
>   for 15 minutes
> 12 clams, scrubbed
> 12 mussels, scrubbed
> 250 g (9 oz) prawns or shrimp, peeled and deveined
> 125 g (4 oz) squid, trimmed and cut into 1 cm (¹/₂ inch) rings (or
>   more shrimp)
> 50 g (2 oz) cooked green peas
> 2 tablespoons finely chopped Italian parsley

1. Heat the olive oil in a shallow, heavy frying pan with a wide mouth (a cast-iron pan that can be brought to the table is ideal). Sauté the onion, garlic and peppers over medium heat until golden brown, 6 minutes, stirring often. Increase the heat to high, add the tomato, and cook for 1 minute. Add the chicken pieces and lightly brown. Transfer the chicken to a plate with tongs and set aside.

2. Add the rice and sauté until the grains are shiny, 1 minute. Add the wine and bring to a boil. Add the stock and saffron and bring to a boil. Reduce the heat and simmer the rice, uncovered, for 10 minutes. Stir in the chicken, clams and mussels, and simmer for 5 minutes. Add the prawns or shrimp and the squid and simmer for 5–8 minutes or until the chicken and seafood are cooked through, the clam and mussel shells have opened, and the rice is tender. Stir in the peas. The paella should be quite moist; if the rice starts to dry out, add a little more stock or water.

3. Just before serving, adjust the seasoning, adding salt and pepper to taste. Sprinkle with the parsley and serve at once.

Makes four servings

PER SERVING: 4 PROTEINS, 2 GRAINS, 1 VEGETABLE, 1 EXTRA

Three-Bean Chilli

Here's a vegetarian chilli that's as colourful as it is tasty. Don't be alarmed by the seemingly large number of ingredients—the recipe can be assembled in 20 minutes, even less if you chop the vegetables in a food processor. If you use canned beans, rinse well to remove excess salt.

    1 tablespoon olive oil
    1 onion, finely chopped
    2 garlic cloves, finely chopped
    1/2 green pepper, finely chopped
    1 jalapeño chilli, seeded and finely chopped
    1 celery stalk, very finely chopped
    1–2 tablespoons chilli powder or to taste
    1/2 teaspoon ground cumin
    1/2 teaspoon dried oregano

200 g (7 oz) cups cooked red kidney beans
200 g (7 oz) cooked cannellini beans
200 g (7 oz) cooked chickpeas
250 g (9 oz) firm tofu, crumbled
400 g (14 oz) can peeled tomatoes, puréed with their juices
250 ml (½ pint) vegetable stock
½ teaspoon Tabasco sauce or to taste
Salt and freshly ground black pepper
1 tablespoon coarse polenta
2 spring onions, chopped, for garnish

1. Heat the olive oil in a large heavy pot. Add onion, garlic, pepper, chilli, and celery and brown over medium heat, about 6 minutes. Add the spices and cook for 1 minute.
2. Stir in the beans, tofu, tomatoes with juices, stock, Tabasco sauce, salt and pepper. Simmer the chilli, uncovered, until thick and flavourful, about 10 minutes. Stir in the polenta in a thin stream to thicken and cook for 1 minute. Adjust the seasoning.
3. To serve, ladle the chilli into bowls and garnish with a sprinkling of spring onions.

Makes four 200 g (7 oz) servings.

Per serving: 4 Proteins, 1 Vegetable, 1 Extra

Teriyaki Salmon with Spicy Slaw

This colourful salmon dish is a favourite at our house. Rice vinegar (available at most supermarkets) has a milder flavour than regular vinegar. If unavailable, use 3 tablespoons distilled white vinegar and 1 tablespoon water. Black sesame seeds, teriyaki sauce and sambal oelek are sold at Asian food shops and good supermarkets.

For the Spicy Slaw
1 garlic clove, minced
1 tablespoon minced fresh ginger
1 spring onion, finely chopped

60 ml (2^1/$_2$ fl oz) rice vinegar
1 tablespoon sugar
^{1}/$_2$ teaspoon sambal oelek (chilli paste)
300 g (11 oz) thinly sliced Chinese or savoy cabbage
^{1}/$_2$ red pepper, thinly sliced
1 carrot, shredded
1 tablespoon black sesame seeds or poppy seeds
Salt and freshly ground black pepper

Teriyaki Salmon

750 g (1^1/$_2$ lb) boneless, skinless salmon fillets, cut into
    four 185g (6 oz) portions
^{1}/$_2$ teaspoon sesame oil or olive oil (on a paper towel)
60 ml (2^1/$_2$ fl oz) teriyaki sauce

1. To make the slaw, in a mixing bowl combine the garlic, ginger, spring onion, vinegar, sugar, and chilli paste. Whisk until the sugar is dissolved. Add the cabbage, pepper, carrot, and sesame seeds and toss to mix. Add salt and pepper to taste.

2. Preheat the grill. Set the top rack about 10 cm (4 inches) below the heat. Lightly oil a baking dish with sesame oil and preheat.

3. Season the fish with salt and pepper and place in the baking dish. Lightly brush the top with teriyaki sauce. Grill the salmon until almost cooked, 6–8 minutes. Brush the remaining teriyaki sauce on the salmon and continue grilling until the fish is cooked through and the top is shiny and brown, 2–4 minutes more.

4. To serve, mound the slaw on plates. Place a piece of fish in the centre of each.

Makes four servings

PER SERVING: 4 PROTEINS, 1 VEGETABLE, 1 EXTRA

Bouillabaisse with Garlic Toasts

Bouillabaisse is the famous Provençal fish stew, brimming with seafood and vegetables, perfumed with orange, and saffron. Once you've assembled the ingredients, this recipe can be prepared in less than 30 minutes. Feel free to vary the seafood, using whatever looks freshest and best at the market.

Bouillabaisse

125 ml (^{1}/$_4$ pint) dry white wine
1 onion, finely chopped
1 leek, washed, trimmed and finely chopped
3 garlic cloves, minced
1 teaspoon dried oregano
1 teaspoon fennel seeds
60 ml (2^1/$_2$ fl oz) fresh orange juice, plus 2 strips of orange zest
1 400 g (14 oz) can peeled tomatoes, puréed with juices
1^1/$_4$ litres (3 pints) defatted chicken or fish stock
250 ml (^{1}/$_4$ pint) water
^{1}/$_2$ teaspoon saffron, soaked in 1 tablespoon hot water for
   15 minutes
2 medium potatoes, peeled and cut into 2^1/$_2$ cm (1 inch) pieces
18 mussels
18 clams or 250 g (^{1}/$_2$ lb) sliced squid
400 g (14 oz) shrimp or prawns, peeled and deveined
400 g (14 oz) skinless, boneless white fish fillets, such as cod or
   snapper, cut into 5 cm (2 inch) pieces
Salt and freshly ground black pepper

For the Garlic Toasts

6 slices French bread, cut diagonally
1 garlic clove, cut in half
2 tablespoons chopped fresh parsley

1. Bring the wine to a boil in a large pot. Add the onion, leek, garlic, oregano, and fennel seeds and simmer briskly until the vegetables are soft, about 3 minutes. Stir in the orange juice and zest and bring to a boil. Add the tomatoes and return to a boil. Transfer this mixture to a food processor or

blender and purée. Return it to the pot. (Or leave the mixture as is—chunky bouillabaisse is delicious too.)

2. Add the stock, water, saffron, and potatoes. Simmer briskly for 5 minutes or until the potatoes are half cooked. Stir in the mussels and clams and simmer for 3 minutes. Stir in the shrimp or prawns and fish and simmer for 5 minutes, or until the potatoes are tender and all the seafood is cooked. Add salt and pepper to taste.

3. Meanwhile, make the garlic toasts. Darkly toast the bread slices in a toaster or under the grill. Transfer to a cake rack to cool. Rub each toast with the cut garlic.

4. To serve the bouillabaisse, ladle the broth and seafood into bowls. Sprinkle with parsley. Place a toast on top of each, half in the bowl, half over the edge, and serve at once.

Makes six servings

PER SERVING: 3 PROTEINS, 1 GRAIN, 2 VEGETABLES

Moroccan Lamb Kebabs

Cumin, coriander and saffron give these kebabs a Moroccan accent. Serve with Lemon Couscous (page 283).

500 g (1 lb) lean leg of lamb, cut into 2¹/₂ cm (1 inch) chunks
¹/₂ teaspoon ground cumin
¹/₂ teaspoon ground coriander
¹/₄ teaspoon saffron threads (crumbled between your fingers)
Salt and freshly ground black pepper
3 tablespoons fresh lemon juice
8 mushrooms
8 pearl onions
8 cherry tomatoes
1 green pepper, cut into 2¹/₂ cm (1 inch) pieces

Garnish
2 tablespoons chopped parsley
1 lemon, quartered

1. Combine the lamb, cumin, coriander, saffron, and salt and pepper in a bowl and toss to mix. Stir in the lemon juice. Marinate for 30 minutes.

2. Preheat the grill to high. Thread the lamb onto skewers, alternating with the mushrooms, onions, cherry tomatoes and pepper pieces. Grill the kebabs until cooked, about 8 minutes in all. Transfer to a platter and sprinkle with parsley. Serve the lemon wedges on the side. Squeeze lemon juice on the kebabs before eating.

Makes four servings

PER SERVING: 4 PROTEINS, 1 VEGETABLE

Spicy Ginger Turkey Stir-Fry

This gingery stir-fry is so full of flavour you won't miss the fat. The recipe uses a technique I call broth-frying: the ingredients are cooked in sizzling stock instead of oil. You can easily create different versions of this recipe by using tofu, chicken or meat instead of turkey and substituting other combinations of vegetables. As with all stir-fries, have all the ingredients chopped, measured out, and ready to go before you start cooking.

For the Sauce

60 ml (2^1/$_2$ fl oz) defatted chicken or vegetable stock, plus 60 ml (2^1/$_2$ fl oz) for stir-frying

2 tablespoons rice wine or sherry

1^1/$_2$ tablespoons soy sauce

1^1/$_2$ tablespoons oyster sauce

2 teaspoons sugar

1 tablespoon cornflour

For the Stir-fry

2 tablespoons minced fresh ginger

3 garlic cloves, minced

3 spring onions, white part minced, green part cut into 2^1/$_2$ cm (1 inch) pieces for garnish

375 g (³/₄ lb) lean turkey breast, sliced into 5 cm (2 inch) long strips
200 g (7 oz) stir-fry vegetables—use a mix of carrots, cabbage, celery and broccoli: the selection and precise amounts of each are flexible

1. To make the sauce, combine the ingredients in a small bowl and stir until the cornflour is dissolved.

2. Just before serving, bring the remaining 60 ml (2¹/₂ fl oz) stock to a boil in a nonstick wok or pan over high heat. Add the ginger, garlic and spring onion whites and stir-fry until fragrant, about 30 seconds. Add the turkey and vegetables and stir-fry until the turkey is almost cooked and the vegetables are almost tender, about 3 minutes. Stir the sauce again to re-dissolve the cornflour and add it to the wok. Continue stir-frying until the turkey is cooked and nicely coated with sauce, 1–2 minutes. Sprinkle with the spring onion greens and serve at once.

Makes four 325 g (12 oz) to 375 (13 oz) servings

PER SERVING: 3 PROTEINS, 1 VEGETABLE

Shabu-Shabu (Japanese Fondue) with Lemon-Ginger Dipping Sauce

Shabu-Shabu is the Japanese version of fondue or Mongolian hot pot. The name is said to echo the sound that the ingredients make as they swish through the broth. The traditional recipe calls for the broth to be flavoured with *kombu* (dried kelp). I've opted for more readily available flavourings, such as ginger and garlic. One of the best things about Shabu-Shabu is that once the ingredients are cooked, you get to enjoy the broth as a soup.

For the Broth
1¹/₂ litres (3 pints) defatted chicken or vegetable stock
4 dried black shiitake mushrooms
2¹/₂ cm (¹/₄ inch) thick fresh ginger slices, flattened with the side of a knife or cleaver
2 garlic cloves, thinly sliced
2 spring onions, thinly sliced

Ingredients for Dipping

    6–8 lettuce leaves, for lining the serving platter

    200 g (7 oz) firm tofu, thinly sliced

    200 g (7 oz) boneless, skinless chicken breast, thinly sliced

    200 g (7 oz) shrimp or prawns, peeled and deveined

    200 g (7 oz) fresh spinach, washed and stemmed

    200 g (7 oz) sliced Chinese or savoy cabbage, cut into 5 cm (2 inch) pieces

    200 g (7 oz) broccoli florets

    4 carrots, very thinly sliced diagonally

    1 large sweet potato, peeled and thinly sliced

For Lemon-Ginger Dipping Sauce

    125 ml ($^1/_4$ pint) fresh lemon juice

    $^1/_2$ teaspoon grated lemon zest

    80 ml (3 fl oz) tamari or substitute soy sauce

    60 ml ($2^1/_2$ fl oz) water

    2 tablespoons sugar

    2 garlic cloves, minced

    2 teaspoons grated fresh ginger

    2 spring onions, finely chopped

    $^1/_4$ teaspoon hot chilli flakes

1. To make the broth, combine the stock, mushrooms, ginger, garlic and spring onions in a fondue pot and simmer for 10 minutes. Remove the mushrooms with a slotted spoon; take off stems and set aside.

2. Line a large platter with lettuce leaves. Arrange the tofu, chicken, shrimp, spinach, Chinese cabbage, broccoli, carrots, sweet potato and mushrooms in neat piles. The Shabu-Shabu can be prepared ahead of this stage and refrigerated.

3. To make the lemon-ginger dipping sauce, combine the ingredients in a bowl and stir to mix.

4. Provide each diner with a plate, a small bowl of dipping sauce, and a set of chopsticks or a fondue fork. Have the broth simmering in a fondue pot (or saucepan on a tabletop burner) in the centre of the table. Have each diner dip the chicken, shrimp or prawns, and vegetables in the simmering broth

and cook them to taste, 1–3 minutes, depending on the ingredient. Since the vegetables—including the decorative lettuce leaves—have come into contact with raw poultry and shrimp, they should not be eaten unless they're first cooked in the broth.

5. After the dipping ingredients are all cooked, take the broth to the kitchen. Season with salt and pepper, strain into bowls, and serve as soup.

Makes four servings

Per serving: 3 Proteins, 2 Vegetables, 1 Extra

Fish en Papillote

Few dishes offer more drama with less preparation time than Fish en Papillote. The fish is baked with vegetables and fresh herbs in an aluminum foil pouch, which seals in all the flavour, creating a great-tasting meal with no added fat. I've called for snapper here, but you could use any fresh fish.

> 2 potatoes (about 500g/1 lb), peeled and thinly sliced
> Salt and freshly ground black pepper
> 4 185 g (6 oz) pieces of snapper or other fish
> 1 tomato, cut into $1/2$ cm ($1/4$ inch) dice
> 1 courgette, cut into $1/2$ cm ($1/4$ inch) dice
> 1 yellow squash, cut into $1/2$ cm ($1/4$ inch) dice
> 1 red pepper, cut into $1/2$ cm ($1/4$ inch) dice
> 4 fresh basil leaves or 1 teaspoon dried basil
> 4 bay leaves
> 125 ml ($1/4$ pint) dry white vermouth or wine

1. Preheat the oven to 200°C (400°F). Arrange four large 5 cm × 8 cm (12 in × 20 in) rectangles of heavy-duty foil on a work surface, shiny side down. In the centre of each, spread out a quarter of the sliced potatoes. Season with salt and pepper. Place a piece of fish on top and season with salt and pepper. Arrange a quarter of the diced tomatoes, courgette, squash, and red pepper, and a basil and a bay leaf on top. Sprinkle with a little more salt and pepper.

2. For each serving, bring together the short edges of the foil rectangle high over the fish. Pour 2 tablespoons of wine over each piece of fish. Crimp the top edges of the foil to form an airtight seal.

3. Place the parcels on baking sheets and bake until the foil is puffed and the fish inside is cooked, about 20 minutes. Serve the parcels on plates. Help each diner open the packet and slide the fish, vegetables and juices onto the plate. Take care not to burn yourselves on the escaping steam.

Makes four servings

Per serving: 3 Proteins, 1 Vegetable

Melon Salad with Yoghurt and Mint

This refreshing fruit salad offers the unexpected flavour combination of ginger and fresh mint.

> 250 ml (½ pint) plain low-fat yoghurt
> ½ teaspoon ground ginger
> ½ teaspoon ground cinnamon
> 2 tablespoons brown sugar
> 2 tablespoons fresh lime juice
> 600 g (1½ lb) cubed cantaloupe or honeydew melon
> 3 tablespoons finely sliced fresh mint leaves,
>   plus 4 whole sprigs for garnish

1. In a mixing bowl, whisk together the yoghurt, ginger, cinnamon, brown sugar and lime juice. Stir in the melon and mint.

2. Transfer the salad to wine glasses or bowls and garnish each with a sprig of fresh mint.

Makes four 200 g (7 oz) servings

Per serving: 1 Fruit, 1 Extra

Orange Custard

This egg-rich dessert might seem like an unlikely candidate for a low-fat makeover. But by using low-fat dairy products and egg whites instead of whole eggs, we can slash the fat to almost nothing. The orange flavour comes through loud and clear thanks to the addition of grated orange zest, orange liqueur, and a perfumed flavouring called orange-flower water. The latter is available in delicatessens. You will need six 180 ml (6 oz) ramekins or custard cups to make the custard.

> 1 440 ml (³/₄ pint) can sweetened low-fat condensed milk
> 300 ml (¹/₂ pint) skimmed milk
> 12 egg whites
> 1 tablespoon Grand Marnier or other orange liqueur
> 1 tablespoon orange-flower water or 1 teaspoon orange extract
> 1 teaspoon vanilla essence
> 1 teaspoon freshly grated orange zest
> ¹/₂ teaspoon ground cinnamon
> A pinch of salt

1. Preheat the oven to 175°C (350°F). Bring 1¹/₄ litres (2¹/₂ pints) of water to the boil.
2. In a mixing bowl, whisk together the condensed milk, skimmed milk, egg whites, orange liqueur, orange-flower water, vanilla, orange zest, cinnamon, and salt. Ladle this mixture into the ramekins. Set the ramekins in a roasting pan, pour 1 cm (¹/₂ inch) boiling water around them, and place in the oven. Bake for 30–40 minutes or until the custards are set. Transfer the custards to a rack to cool, then refrigerate for at least 4 hours, preferably overnight. Serve cold.

Makes six servings

PER SERVING: 1 DAIRY, 1 PROTEIN, 2 EXTRAS

Coconut Fruit Salad

Toasted coconut adds a tropical touch to this colourful fruit salad. You can replace any of the fruits mentioned below with other fruits in season.

1 starfruit, thinly sliced
1 banana, peeled and diced
2 kiwifruits, peeled and diced

150 g (5 oz) fresh blueberries
1 orange, peeled and cut or broken into segments
2 tablespoons coconut rum (such as Malibu) or orange liqueur
2 tablespoons coconut, lightly toasted

1. Set 4 starfruit slices aside for garnish. (Make a slit in each so it will slip over the edge of a glass.) Combine the remaining fruit and rum in a mixing bowl and gently toss to mix.
2. Spoon the fruit into wine or martini glasses and sprinkle each with with a little toasted coconut. Slide a starfruit slice over the edge of each glass and serve at once.
Note: To toast your own coconut, buy sweetened grated coconut in the supermarket and toast it in a thin layer on a baking sheet in a 200°C (400°F) oven until golden brown, about 5 minutes.

Makes four 250 g (9 oz) servings

P ER SERVING: 1 F RUIT, 1 E XTRA

Blueberry Soup

Here's a colourful soup that's as refreshing as it is unexpected. You can use frozen berries if the fresh are unavailable.

225 g (8 oz) fresh blueberries
250 ml (½ pint) cranberry juice
375 ml (⅔ pint) water
90 ml (3 fl oz) white wine
1 tablespoon sugar or to taste
2 teaspoons minced fresh ginger

1 cinnamon stick
2 teaspoons cornflour
90 ml (3 fl oz) port
8 fresh mint leaves, thinly sliced

1. Pick through the berries, removing any stems. Wash well. Place the berries, cranberry juice, water, white wine, sugar, ginger and cinnamon in a pot and bring to a boil. Simmer the blueberries for 5 minutes.

2. Dissolve the cornflour in the port and whisk the mixture into the berries. Simmer for 3 minutes. Discard the cinnamon stick and purée the soup in a blender. Or leave the soup chunky if you prefer. Transfer to a bowl and allow to cool to room temperature, then refrigerate until cold. If too thick, thin with a little water.

3. To serve, ladle the soup into wine goblets or brandy snifters. Sprinkle the mint on top and serve.

Makes four servings

PER SERVING: 1 FRUIT, 1 EXTRA

Strawberry Napoleons

Here's a stunning dessert for entertaining that has only a fraction of the fat found in the traditional recipe. The secret is to use a baked wonton wrapper to make the pastry. Wonton wrappers are available in Asian food shops. Or use egg roll wrappers, cutting them into 7½ cm (3 inch) squares. Don't be intimidated by the length of the recipe. It's really just a series of simple steps.

For the Pastry
Oil cooking spray
12 wonton wrappers, each about 7½ cm (3 inch) square
4 teaspoons sugar
½ teaspoon cinnamon

For the Pastry Cream
250 ml (½ pint) skimmed milk
3 tablespoons granulated sugar

$1^1/2$ tablespoons cornflour

1 egg

1 teaspoon orange liqueur

$^1/2$ teaspoon vanilla essence

$^1/2$ teaspoon grated lemon zest

To finish the napoleons

1 kg (2 lb) strawberries

1 tablespoon icing sugar

1. To make the pastry, first preheat the oven to 200°C (400°F). Lightly spray a non-stick baking sheet with oil. Arrange the wonton wrappers on top and lightly spray with oil. Mix the 4 teaspoons of sugar and cinnamon in a small bowl and lightly sprinkle this mixture over the wonton wrappers. Bake until golden brown and crisp, about 5 minutes. Transfer the wrappers to a cake rack to cool. The pastry tastes best served within 2 hours of being baked. If you wish to prepare the wrappers ahead of time or even the day before store them in an airtight tin to keep them from getting soggy.

2. To prepare the pastry cream, heat the milk in a saucepan and gradually bring to a boil, stirring often to prevent scorching. In a mixing bowl, whisk together the remaining 3 tablespoons of sugar and cornflour. Add the egg and whisk to mix. Whisk the scalded milk into the egg mix in a thin stream. Return to the pan and bring to a boil, whisking steadily.

3. Reduce the heat and cook the cream until thickened, about 2 minutes. The mixture should bubble. Transfer the pastry cream to a bowl and whisk in the orange liqueur, vanilla essence and lemon zest. Press a piece of plastic wrap on top of the cream to prevent a skin from forming, making a slit in the top to allow the steam to escape. Let cool to room temperature, then refrigerate until cold. The cream can be made up to 24 hours ahead.

4. Not more than 1 hour before serving, wash, stem, and thinly slice half the strawberries. Leave the remaining berries whole for decoration.

5. Shortly before serving, excuse yourself from the table and assemble the napoleons in the kitchen. (Better yet, invite everyone into the kitchen to watch!) Arrange 4 baked wonton wrappers on a work surface. Gently spread a couple of tablespoons of pastry cream on each wrapper and arrange the strawberry slices on top. (You should use up half the pastry cream and sliced berries.) Place a second wonton wrapper on top and top with the remaining pastry cream and berries. Place a third wonton wrapper on top. Sift a little

icing sugar over each napoleon. Using a spatula, transfer the napoleons to plates. Garnish with the whole berries and serve.

Makes four servings

PER SERVING: 1 GRAIN, 1 FRUIT, 2 EXTRAS

Peaches in Sparkling Wine

    1 ripe peach
    185 ml ($^1/_3$ pint) sparkling wine

Dice 1 ripe peach into a wineglass. Fill the glass with sparkling wine.

Makes one serving

PER SERVING: 1 FRUIT, 1 EXTRA

Indian Milk Shake

Lassi is the Indian version of a milk shake, a refreshing, nourishing beverage made with yoghurt, ice, and rose water, a perfumed flavouring popular in Indian and Middle Eastern cooking. Look for it at delicatessens and at your local pharmacy.

    250 ml ($^1/_2$ pint) plain low-fat yoghurt
    2 teaspoons honey or to taste
    $^1/_2$ teaspoon rose water or to taste
    4 ice-cubes
    $^1/_8$ teaspoon ground cardamom

1. Combine the yoghurt, honey, rose water and ice in a blender and blend until smooth. Adjust the seasoning, adding honey or rose water to taste.
2. Pour *lassi* into a tall glass. Sprinkle cardamom on top and serve at once.

Makes one serving

PER SERVING: 1 DAIRY, 1 EXTRA

Fruit Juice Spritzer

100 ml (¼ pint) fruit juice
185 ml (⅓ pint) sparkling mineral water

Combine fruit juice with mineral water.

Makes one serving

Per serving: ½ Fruit

Lemon-Mint Spritzer

1 tablespoon lemon juice
Lemon slice
Mineral water
Fresh mint

Add lemon juice and a lemon slice to a glass of mineral water. Add a bruised sprig of fresh mint.

Makes one serving

Per serving: Next to Nothing

Peach Yoghurt Smoothie

1 peach
250 ml (½ pint) plain low-fat yoghurt
2 teaspoons honey
4 ice-cubes

Purée peach, yoghurt, honey, and ice-cubes in a blender. Serve immediately.

Makes one serving

Per serving: 1 Fruit, 1 Dairy, 1 Extra

Vietnamese Iced Coffee

1 cup ice
1 tablespoon sweetened low-fat condensed milk
250 ml (½ pint) hot coffee

Fill a tall glass with ice. Add the condensed milk. Place a spoon in the glass. Slowly add the hot coffee, pouring it on the spoon to absorb the heat.

Makes one serving

PER SERVING: 1 EXTRA

Café de Olla

Café de Olla is spice-flavoured Mexican coffee.

250 ml (½ pint) hot coffee
A pinch of ground cinnamon
A pinch of ground clove
2 teaspoons brown sugar
½ teaspoon vanilla essence

To a cup of your favourite coffee, add the cinnamon, clove, brown sugar and vanilla.

Makes one serving

PER SERVING: 1 EXTRA

Café Latte

60 ml (2¹/₂ fl oz) espresso or strong coffee
250 ml (¹/₂ pint) hot skimmed milk

Combine the espresso with the hot milk.

Makes one serving

PER SERVING: 1 DAIRY

Mexican Scrambled Egg

Serve this with your favourite salsa. If you like spicy food, leave the chilli seeds in.

4 flour tortillas or pitta bread
4 teaspoons olive oil
1 onion, finely chopped
2 garlic cloves, finely chopped
1–2 jalapeño chillies, seeded and finely chopped
1 tomato, seeded and finely chopped
3 sprigs chopped fresh coriander
12 egg whites, lightly beaten
Salt and freshly ground black pepper
75g (3 oz) of your favourite salsa

1. Cut each tortilla or pitta into 8 wedges. Place on a baking sheet and cook in a preheated 200°C (400°F) oven until golden brown, about 5 minutes. Transfer to a rack and let cool.
2. Heat the oil in a non-stick frying pan. Add the onion, garlic and chillies and cook until the onion is soft but not brown, about 4 minutes. Add the tomato and half the coriander and cook for 2 minutes. Add the eggs, salt and pepper to taste and cook until scrambled, about 3 minutes. Adjust the seasoning if necessary.

3. Serve the scrambled eggs with the tortilla chips and salsa.

Makes one serving

Per serving: 1 Protein, 1 Grain, 1 Vegetable, 1 Extra

Cinnamon-Orange Popovers

Cinnamon, orange zest, and almond extract add so much flavour to these popovers that you won't miss the egg yolks and butter found in traditional recipes. The secret to achieving a dramatic puff is to bake the popovers in deep non-stick moulds.

> 250 g (9 oz) unbleached plain flour
> $1/2$ teaspoon ground cinnamon
> $1/2$ teaspoon freshly grated orange zest
> $1/2$ teaspoon almond essence
> $1/2$ teaspoon salt
> 250 ml ($1/2$ pint) skimmed milk, at room temperature
> 4 egg whites
> 2 teaspoons canola oil or melted butter

1. Preheat the oven to 230°C (450°F). Lightly spray or wipe the moulds with oil.
2. Combine all the ingredients in a blender and mix until smooth. Pour the batter into the moulds, filling each mould a third of the way.
3. Bake the popovers for 15 minutes without opening the oven door. Lower the heat to 175°C (350°F) and continue baking for 30 minutes, or until the popovers are puffed and well browned. Unmould and serve at once.
Note: If you don't own moulds, use muffin tins, filling each about halfway. Alternatively, you can bake the batter in a baking dish in the style of Yorkshire pudding.

Makes 6 large popovers, one per serving

Per serving: 1 Grain, 1 Extra

Cream of Wheat Cereal

375 ml (²/₃ pint) skimmed milk
70 ml (2½ fl oz) cream of wheat
A pinch of salt
2 teaspoons blueberry syrup

1. Slowly heat the milk until it reaches a simmer.
2. Stir in cream of wheat and salt. Simmer for about 3 minutes, stirring until the cereal thickens.
3. Serve with blueberry syrup.

Makes one serving

Per serving: 1½ Dairy (or count as 1 Dairy and 1 Protein), 2 Grains, 1 Extra

Muesli Parfait

This takes just seconds to make, but it really looks terrific. Remember, we eat with our eyes as well as our palates.

50 g (2 oz) low-fat plain muesli
250 ml (½ pint) low-fat plain yoghurt
40 g (1½ oz) blueberries

In a parfait glass or wine glass, layer the muesli, yoghurt and blueberries.

Makes one serving

Per serving: 1 Dairy, 1 Grain, ½ Fruit

INDEX

▼　　▼　　▼　　▼

ABOUT MIRIAM E. NELSON, Ph.D. AND SARAH WERNICK, Ph.D.

Authors of *Strong Women Stay Slim* and the international bestseller *Strong Women Stay Young*

Miriam E. Nelson, Ph.D., is Associate Chief of the Human Physiology Laboratory at the Jean Mayer USDA Human Nutrition Research Center on Aging at Tufts University and Assistant Professor at the School of Nutrition Science and Policy. She is a Fellow of the American College of Sports Medicine and holds their certification as a health/fitness director. Her original research papers have been published in distinguished peer-reviewed journals, including the *Journal of the American Medical Association* and the *New England Journal of Medicine*. She is a former Brookdale National Fellow and is currently a Bunting Fellow at Radcliffe College.

Sarah Wernick, Ph.D., is an award-winning freelance writer based in Brookline, Massachusetts. Her articles have appeared in *Woman's Day*, *Working Mother*, *Smithsonian*, the *New York Times*, and other publications.

The *Strong Women* World Wide Web site is
http://www.strongwomen.com

Also by Miriam E. Nelson, Ph.D.
with Sarah Wernick, Ph.D.

Strong Women
Stay Young

Reduce loss of bone density, gain more energy, and look and feel ten to fifteen years younger!

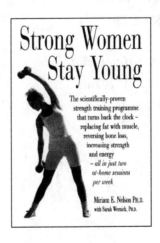

This scientifically proven strength-training programme turns back the clock for women aged 35 and up – replacing fat with muscle, increasing strength and energy, improving balance and flexibility – all in just two sessions per week. Research by Dr Nelson created worldwide news when the results were published in the *Journal of the American Medical Association* in 1994. Her study showed that after a year of strength training twice a week women's bodies were 15–20 years more youthful.

Without drugs, they regained bone, helping to prevent osteoporosis; they became stronger, leaner and trimmer, and were so energised they became 27% more active.

Aurum Press   ISBN 1 85410 498 5

Other health titles available from Aurum Press

Strong Women Stay Young
Miriam E. Nelson Ph.D. with Sarah Wernick Ph.D.
ISBN 1 85410 498 5

Smart Exercise
Covert Bailey
ISBN 1 85410 311 3

Body Learning
An Introduction to the Alexander Texhnique
Michael Gelb
ISBN 1 85410 286 9

Understanding Childbirth
Betty Parsons MBE
ISBN 1 85410 412 8